HASHIMOTO DIET

HASHIMOTO BE GONE!

The Complete Meal Plan To Heal Your Body From Hypothyroidism and Throiditis

Amber Copeland

from the Publisher. All additional right reserved.

The information in the following pages is broadly considered to be a truthful and accurate account of facts and as such any inattention, use or misuse of the information in question by the reader will render any resulting actions solely under their purview. There are no scenarios in which the publisher or the original author of this work can be in any fashion deemed liable for any hardship or damages that may befall them after undertaking information described herein.

Additionally, the information in the following pages is intended only for informational purposes and should thus be thought of as universal. As befitting its nature, it is presented without assurance regarding its prolonged validity or interim quality. Trademarks that are mentioned are done without written consent and can in no way be considered an endorsement from the trademark holder.

Table of Contents

PART I

Hashimoto Diet

This chapter will give you a brief introduction to what the Hashimoto disease is and what diet you can follow in this case.

Chapter 1: Causes and Symptoms of Hashimoto Disease

Hashimoto's disease is a type of autoimmune disorder. It may lead to hypothyroidism (i.e., underactive thyroid). When you have this disease, your thyroid gets attacked by your immune system. It causes immense damage to the thyroid gland as a result of which it fails to produce an adequate amount of thyroid hormones. Hashimoto's disease causes inflammation (chronic lymphocytic thyroiditis), which eventually leads to hypothyroidism. Men and women of all ages and even children can get affected by this disease. Middle-aged women are more likely to get affected by this particular disease. Generally, a thyroid function test is suggested by the doctors for the detection of Hashimoto's disease. This disease can be treated by a simple thyroid hormone replacement effectively.

A study stated that earlier, it was a little difficult for the doctors to detect Hashimoto's disease. But now it can be easily identified by an antibody test (since this disease causes the production of harmful antibodies) and a hormone test (during hypothyroidism, the thyroid hormone level is low, whereas the level of TSH is more). The pituitary glands release more TSH so that it can stimulate the thyroid to increase the production of the thyroid hormone.

Causes of Hashimoto's Disease

- People who get exposed to enormous amounts of radiation are more likely to develop Hashimoto's disease.

- Having an underlying medical condition often acts as a triggering factor in the case of developing new health issues. If you already have an autoimmune disease like type-1 diabetes or rheumatoid arthritis, then you are more prone to Hashimoto's disease.

- Heredity is an important factor when it comes to autoimmune diseases. So, if there is Hashimoto's disease in your family history, then you have a fair chance of developing the same.

- People of all ages can get affected by Hashimoto's disease, but middle-aged people are at higher risk.

- Gender is also a factor as women are more prone to this particular disease.

Symptoms of Hashimoto's Disease

Hashimoto's disease can be asymptomatic at the beginning, but it slowly starts showing you symptoms after a few days. Let's see some of the symptoms of this disease.

- Memory lapse

- Depression

- Heavy menstrual bleeding (can also be prolonged)

- Muscle fatigue

- Pain in the joints and stiffness

- Muscle aches, stiffness, and tenderness

- Uncontrollable weight gain

- Tongue enlargement

- Loss of hair

- Nails become brittle

- The face becomes puffed up

- Dry and pale skin

- Constipation

- Hypersensitivity to cold

- Sluggishness and fatigue

Supplements That You Can Take

Millions of individuals are surviving in this world who is suffering from Hashimoto's Disease or Hashimoto thyroiditis. This deep-rooted autoimmune situation makes the thyroid gland inactive. It is true that Hashimoto Disease develops or progresses slowly. But, such autoimmune condition attacks as well as destroys the thyroid gland. The symptoms of this disease might remain unnoticed for many years. Treatment begins after checking levels of one-two antibodies, namely thyroglobulin (Tg) and thyroperoxidase (TPO). In certain cases, the thyroid gland might also be checked through ultrasound. But, you need not worry as you may survive well even with this disease. Besides medical intervention, various supplements are available that play a crucial role in dealing with Hashimoto Disease.

But, before consuming any such supplements, it is better to consult your healthcare provider or practitioner. He or she is the perfect person who will be able to guide you according to your health condition. Here you will get to know about some of the essential supplements that you may consume for Hashimoto Disease.

- **Selenium**- Selenium assists the thyroid gland in producing thyroid hormone. It is also helpful in converting T4 (thyroxine) into T3 (triiodothyronine). Various studies have revealed the fact that selenium supplementation is effective for treating this disease, whether combined with levothyroxine or used alone. Selenium supplements are beneficial, but it is better not to consume more than one hundred micrograms (mcg) each day. You may intake more or less than the mentioned quantity only if your doctor prescribes you to do so. For more trust-worthy selenium consumption, it is better to rely on supplements than food sources.

- **Zinc**- In accordance with certain reliable research, supplementation of zinc might help maintain a healthy thyroid hormone level. Expert healthcare providers usually suggest fifteen to thirty mg of zinc supplement daily. Zinc and selenium together are worthy of improving the functioning of the thyroid.

- **Omega-3 Fatty Acid**- It is believed that omega-3 fatty acids, particularly docosahexaenoic acid (DHA) and icosapentaenoic acid (EPA) are helpful for individual suffering from autoimmune thyroid conditions. It is recommended to consume fish oil supplements twice or thrice a week. Omega-3 fatty acid supplement (plant-based) is also beneficial but is not so well absorbed like fish oil supplements.

- **Vitamin B1**- Evidence exists that thiamine or vitamin B1 supplements are useful in reducing fatigue of those people having Hashimoto's thyroiditis. This disease leads to decreased thiamine absorption. If you are facing such a problem, you may discuss it with your physician for the dosage of thiamine supplementation.

Chapter 2: Recipes for Appetizers and Snacks

Oven Roasted Okra

Total Prep & Cooking Time: 35 minutes

Yields: Four servings

Nutrition Facts: Calories: 104 | Carbs: 9.4g | Protein: 2.2g | Fat: 7.2g | Fiber: 3.6g

Ingredients:

- One pound of okra
- One tbsp. each of
  - Lemon juice
  - Balsamic vinegar
- One teaspoon each of
  - Onion powder
  - Garlic powder
- A quarter teaspoon of black pepper
- Two tablespoons of avocado oil
- A three-fourth teaspoon of sea salt

Method:

1. Set the oven temperature at 400 degrees F. You will require a baking sheet to bake the okra. With a parchment paper, line the sheet.

2. Rinse the okras thoroughly under running water and dry them. Chop off the head of each okra. Slice each okra into five pieces and then set them aside.

3. Place the okra pieces evenly on the sheet and top them with salt, pepper, lemon, oil, and balsamic vinegar. Toss them well so that the okra is entirely coated with the seasonings.

4. Transfer the sheet to an oven and roast them for twenty-four to twenty-five minutes. Flip the pieces in between to cook both sides evenly.

5. Take the sheet off the oven and then allow them to cool down.

6. Serve and enjoy.

Note: *Okra is an incredibly delicious summer vegetable.*

Honeydew Smoothie Bowl

Total Prep & Cooking Time: 5 minutes

Yields: 2 servings

Nutrition Facts: Calories: 176 | Carbs: 41.4g | Protein: 2.5g | Fat: 1.6g | Fiber: 3g

Ingredients:

- One tbsp. of honey
- One-third cup of green juice of your choice (for example, wheatgrass)
- Half a cup of coconut milk beverage (unsweetened)
- Four cups of cubed honeydew (frozen, make pieces of half an inch in size)
- Salt as per taste
- For garnishing – nuts, fresh basil, berries, and melon balls

Method:

1. Use a high-speed blender or food processor to blend the following ingredients together – salt, honey, juice, coconut milk, and honeydew. Stop in between blending and pulsing to scrape down the sides of the food processor.

2. Pulse for about one to two minutes to get your desired consistency. Before serving, top the smoothie with toppings of your choice.

Wake-Up Smoothie

Total Prep & Cooking Time: 5 minutes

Yields: 3 servings

Nutrition Facts: Calories: 139 | Carbs: 28g | Protein: 4.4g | Fat: 2g | Fiber: 4.3g

Ingredients:

- One banana
- 1.25 cups of orange juice (if possible, then calcium-fortified)
- Half a cup of silken tofu (low-fat) or low-fat yogurt
- 1.25 cups of frozen berries such as blackberries, raspberries, strawberries, or blueberries
- One tbsp. of sugar or Stevia

Method:

1. In the bowl of a blender, add the ingredients.
2. Cover the bowl and blend the ingredients until you get a smooth and creamy mixture.
3. Serve and enjoy!

Cucumber Radish Salsa

Total Prep Time: 10 minutes

Yields: Four plates of salsa

Nutrition Facts: Calories: 22 | Carb: 4.7g | Protein: 0.9g | Fat: 0.4g | Fiber: 1.6g

Ingredients:

- One large-sized cucumber (sliced)
- A quarter cup of chopped cilantro
- Two juiced limes
- One heaping cup of radishes, eight to ten regular (either sliced into thin halves or diced)
- Three tablespoons of diced red onion
- One tablespoon of olive oil
- To taste: Pepper (freshly ground and optional) and salt

Method:

1. In a bowl, place all the veggies listed in the ingredients section.

2. Combine them thoroughly, and place them in a refrigerator for one hour before serving.

Crispy Oven-Fried Fish Tacos

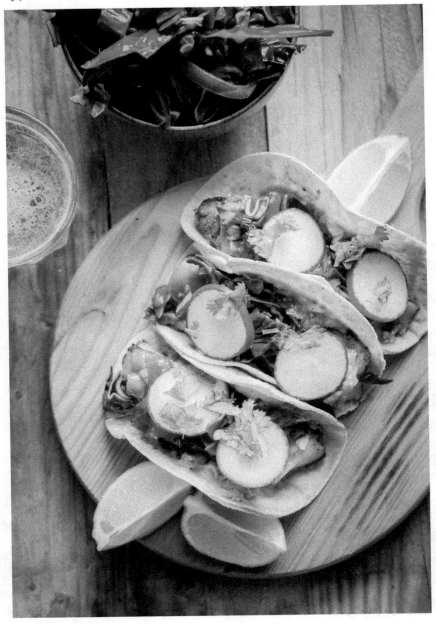

Total Prep & Cooking Time: 45 minutes

Yields: 4 servings (Two tacos per serving)

Nutrition Facts: Calories: 496 | Carbs: 65.4g | Protein: 27.3g | Fat: 17.6g | Fiber: 15.2g

Ingredients:

- A cup of cereal flakes (whole-grain)
- Cooking spray
- Half a tsp. each of
    - Salt (keep it divided)
    - Paprika
    - Garlic powder
- Half a cup of all-purpose flour
- Three-quarter tsp. of freshly ground pepper (keep it divided)
- Three-quarter cups of breadcrumbs (whole wheat)
- Two egg whites
- One lb. of cod (cut into strips)
- Two tbsps. each of
    - Avocado oil
    - Water
    - Unseasoned rice vinegar
- One avocado (sliced)
- Pico de gallo
- Three cups of coleslaw mix
- Eight warmed corn tortillas

Method:

1. Set the temperature of the oven to 450 degrees F and preheat. Take a baking sheet and, on it, place a wire rack. Use cooking spray to coat it nicely.

2. In the bowl of a food processor, add the breadcrumbs, cereal flakes, paprika, garlic powder, half a tsp. of pepper, and half a tsp. of salt. Process all these ingredients until you get a smooth mixture. Take this mixture and spread it on a shallow dish.

3. Take another shallow dish and place flour on it. Then, in the third shallow dish, whisk water and egg together.

4. Take each fillet of fish, dredge it in flour, and then dip the fillet in the egg mixture. Then, coat both sides of the fillets with breadcrumbs evenly.

5. Once done, place these fillets on the greased wire racks. The breaded fish should be coated with cooking spray as well. Bake them for about ten minutes by the end of which they should become golden brown and crispy.

6. Meanwhile, take a medium-sized bowl and, in it, whisk the following ingredients together – remaining pepper and salt, vinegar, and oil. Add the mix of coleslaw to it and toss nicely so that everything is evenly coated.

7. Finally, take the tortillas, divide the avocados, coleslaw mix, and fish evenly. If you want, then serve them with pico de gallo.

Strawberry Mango Salsa

Total Prep Time: 10 minutes

Yields: Four servings

Nutrition Facts: Calories: 126 | Carbs: 20.3g | Protein: 1.8g | Fat: 5.7g | Fiber: 4.6g

Ingredients:

- One cup of diced strawberries
- A quarter cup of diced red onions
- A tablespoon of chopped cilantro
- One medium-sized mango (chopped)
- One medium avocado (sliced)
- One lime, juiced
- To taste: Salt

Method:

1. In a bowl (medium-sized), add all ingredients listed in the section, except the salt. Carefully combine them with spatula's help so that the veggies get well coated with the lime juice. Make sure that you do not crush the avocado pieces.

2. After the ingredients have been entirely tossed, sprinkle over the salt. You can serve immediately, or you can store in the refrigerator in a closed container.

Strawberry Mousse

Total Prep & Cooking Time: 6 hours and 30 minutes

Yields: Six servings

Nutrition Facts: Calories: 100 | Carbs: 20g | Protein: 5g | Fat: 0g | Fiber: 1g

Ingredients:

- Twelve ounces of halved and hulled fresh strawberries
- A three-fourth cup of Greek yogurt
- Lemon juice (few drops)
- One-third cup of honey
- Four egg whites
- Salt to taste

Method:

1. Place strawberries and honey in a blender and make them smooth. Put them in a bowl.

2. Pour the yogurt in the bowl and whisk them properly.

3. Take another bowl. Add the lemon splash, salt, and egg whites. Using a hand mixer, whisk the eggs to form stiff peaks such a way that the egg remains intact when turned upside down.

4. With a spatula, mix one-third of the egg mixture with strawberry. Slowly pour the rest of the egg whites mixture, ensuring that the bubbles do not break.

5. Transfer to six containers. Store the containers for six hours in the refrigerator. Enjoy.

Grilled Salmon and Veggies

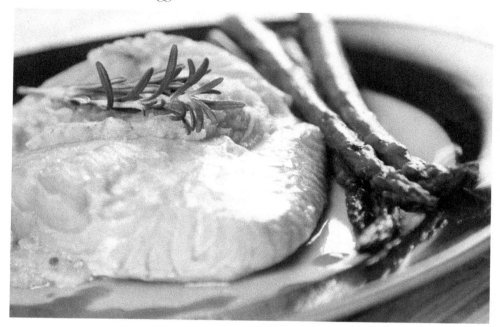

Total Prep & Cooking Time: 25 minutes

Yields: Four servings

Nutrition Facts: Calories: 281 | Carbs: 10.6g | Protein: 30.2g | Fat: 2.3g | Fiber: 3.1g

Ingredients:

- One medium-sized zucchini, sliced vertically into halves
- One onion (cut into wedges of one-inch), red

- Half a tsp. of salt
- One and a quarter lb. of salmon fillets (sliced into portions of four)
- One lemon, sliced into wedges of four
- Two bell peppers (each of red, orange, yellow), halved, seeded, and trimmed
- One tbsp. of olive oil (extra-virgin)
- Half a tsp. of pepper (ground)
- A quarter cup of fresh basil (thinly sliced)

Method:

1. Keep the grill preheated to moderate heat.

2. Place onions, pepper, and zucchini in a bowl sprinkle some salt (a quarter tsp.) and brush them with oil.

3. Place the salmon fillets in another bowl and sprinkle with remaining salt and pepper.

4. Transfer the salmon and the veggies to grill and then cook the vegetables occasionally, turning and cooking each side for six minutes until they tenderize. Cook the salmon for ten minutes until they flake.

5. Remove the vegetables and chop them into small pieces when they have cooled down. Toss them well. Serve the salmon aside the vegetables. Garnish them with one tbsp. of basil and the lemon wedges.

Chapter 3: Main Course Recipes

Zucchini Noodles With Shrimp and Avocado Pesto

Total Prep & Cooking Time: 35 minutes

Yields: 4 servings (1.75 cups each serving)

Nutrition Facts: Calories: 446 | Carbs: 15.8g | Protein: 25.9g | Fat: 33.2g | Fiber: 6.6g

Ingredients:

- One avocado (ripe)
- One cup of basil leaves (fresh)
- Three-quarter tsp. of salt (keep it divided)
- Five-six zucchini (medium-sized, trimmed)
- A quarter cup of pistachios (shelled, unsalted)
- Three garlic cloves (minced)
- A quarter cup of olive oil (extra-virgin variety, + two tbsps. extra)
- A quarter tsp. of freshly ground pepper
- 1-2 tsps. of Old Bay seasoning
- One lb. of raw shrimp (deveined and peeled)
- Two tbsps. of lemon juice

Method:

1. Your first step is to prepare the zucchini using a spiralizer and form thin strips. Then, take the zoodles and place them in a colander. Sprinkle half a tsp. of salt. Allow it to drain for half an hour and squeeze to remove any excess water.

2. In a food processor, combine the following – pepper, lemon juice, pistachios basil, avocado, and a quarter tsp. of salt. Make sure everything is finely chopped. To make it smooth, add a quarter cup of oil.

3. In a large-sized skillet, heat one tbsp. of oil on medium-high flame. Cook the garlic in the heated oil for about thirty seconds. Then, sprinkle the Old Bay seasoning and add the shrimp. Keep stirring and cook the shrimp for about four minutes. Once done, transfer the shrimp to a bowl.

4. Take the remaining one tbsp. of oil and add it to the pan. The zoodles should have drained by now, so you have to add them to the pan and toss them for about three minutes. Then, transfer them to the bowl containing shrimp and mix properly. Add the pesto and combine it by tossing everything once again. Serve and enjoy!

Honey Ginger Shrimp Bowls

Total Prep & cooking Time: 26 minutes

Yields: Two bowls

Nutrition Facts: Calories: 165.9 | Carbs: 4.1g | Protein: 19g | Fat: 8.1g | Fiber: 0.8g

Ingredients:

For preparing the shrimp,

- Twelve ounces of large deveined and peeled shrimp (uncooked)
- One teaspoon of freshly minced ginger
- Two teaspoons of avocado oil
- Two tablespoons each of
  - o Honey
  - o Coconut aminos
- Two cloves of garlic (diced)
- To taste: salt, lime, pepper (ground freshly, optional)

Dressing ingredients,

- Two tablespoons each of
  - o Olive oil
  - o Lime juice
- A quarter teaspoon each of

- o Ginger powder
- o Garlic powder
- One teaspoon each of
  - o Coconut aminos
  - o Honey
- To taste – Pepper and salt

Salad ingredients,

- Four cups of spinach or arugula
- Four onions sliced (green)
- One avocado (diced)
- Half a cup each of
  - o Carrots (shredded)
  - o Radishes (shredded)
- A quarter of cilantro (sliced)

Method:

1. Take a bowl and put coconut aminos, ginger, honey, and garlic. Combine them well with a whisk.

2. Take a lidded container and pour the shrimp into it along with the marinade. Stir thoroughly.

3. Marinate the shrimp for two hours in the refrigerator.

4. After the period described above, pour some avocado oil in the skillet and heat over moderate flame. Pour the shrimp mixture into the skillet. Cook for about three minutes to make the shrimp opaque and then flip.

5. Continue cooking for an additional three minutes to make the sauce thickened—season with lime, pepper, and salt. Cook well to form an even coating over the shrimp pieces.

6. Toss carrots, greens, and radishes in a bowl and then divide equally into two plates.

7. To serve: top each dish with the cooked shrimp, cilantro, avocado, dressing, onions, and wedges.

Note: You can chop the carrots and radishes with shredding attachment or the box grater. Be careful while cooking the shrimp. The inner flesh must be white, and the outer tissue should turn pink.

Beef and Sweet Potatoes Stew

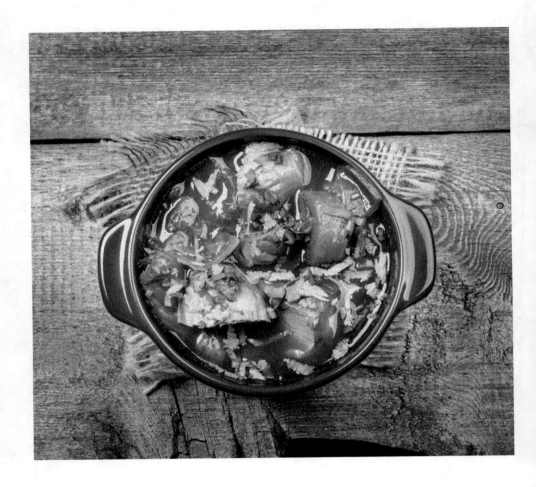

Total Prep & Cooking Time: 20 minutes

Yields: Four servings

Nutrition Facts: Calories: 195 | Carbs: 18g | Protein: 19g | Fat: 5g | Fiber: 3g

Ingredients:

- One teaspoon each of
  - Avocado oil
  - Salt
- One tablespoon of minced ginger
- Two teaspoons each of
  - Oregano (dried)
  - Thyme (dried)
- One cup each of
  - Pumpkin puree
  - Cilantro (chopped)
  - Carrots (sliced)
- One pound of grass-fed beef (ground)
- Diced avocado
- One diced onion
- Three cloves of garlic (minced)
- Five cups of cubed and peeled sweet potato
- Two cups bone broth
- Two limes juiced
- Six sliced green onions
- Pepper to taste and optional

Method:

1. Pour avocado oil in an instant pot and set the function to 'saute.' After oil starts to boil, add the ginger, carrots, onion, garlic, sweet potatoes, thyme, pepper, salt, and oregano, stir for few minutes until you get the smell.

2. Turn it off. Add the bone broth and the pumpkin puree to the mixture and beef (ground) to form a single layer at the bottom.

3. Cook the stew using the manual setting for five minutes. Release the method by switching to the quick-release mode.

4. Season with lime juice. Divide equally among four bowls and top with avocado and herbs to serve.

Roasted Sunchoke Salad

Total Prep & Cooking Time: 35 minutes

Yields: Four servings

Nutrition Facts: Calories: 143 | Carbs: 20g | Protein: 2g | Fat: 6g | Fiber: 2g

Ingredients:

- Two pounds of trimmed and scrubbed sunchokes
- Half a cup of minced red onion
- Two tablespoons of avocado oil
- A three-fourth cup of parsley (minced)
- One clove of garlic (diced)
- To taste: Black pepper (ground) and salt

Method:

1. Set the oven at a temperature of 425 degrees F. place a baking sheet on your countertop. Mix the sunchokes, pepper, salt, and one tbsp. of avocado oil. Toss them well over the baking sheet in an even layer.

2. Bake for thirty minutes, occasionally stirring until the edges turn brown and crispy, leaving the middle portions creamy.

3. Meanwhile, in a bowl, place the remaining ingredients and then add the sunchokes mixture. Stir them well and add some seasoning if required.

4. Serve immediately.

Kale Salad

Total Prep Time: 20 minutes

Yields: Four bowls of salad

Nutrition Facts: Calories: 334 | Carbs: 19g | Protein: 9g | Fat: 26g | Fiber: 4g

Ingredients:

- Five cups of chopped kale
- One-eighth tsp. of salt
- Half a cup each of
  o Cheese
  o Sliced almonds
- A quarter cup each of
  o Seeds of sunflower
  o Cranberries
  o Diced red onions
- Two tsps. of olive oil
- Two cups of chopped broccoli
- A quarter to a half cup of shredded carrots

For the lemon dressing,

- A quarter cup of oil (olive)
- One tbsp. of Dijon mustard
- Half a tsp. of oregano (dried)

- One-eighth tsp. of black pepper (ground)
- Two tbsps. each of
  - Lemon juice
  - Vinegar (red wine)
- One garlic clove (minced)
- A quarter tsp. of salt
- One tsp. of sugar or honey

Method:

1. Massage the chopped kale leaves with salt and oil. Brush them with the fingers to make the leaves become tender and darken in color.

2. For the dressing, mix all ingredients in the jar with a lid. Shake them well so that they emulsify. Adjust the sweetener, pepper, and salt as your heart desires.

3. Take a bowl and place broccoli, massaged kale, cheese, onion, almond, carrots, cranberries, and sunflower seeds. Toss them well. Pour the dressing ingredients over it (about one-third). Shake well to coat and then add the extra dressing according to your taste.

Taco Spaghetti Squash Boats

Total Prep & Cooking Time: 45 minutes

Yields: Four servings

Nutrition Facts: Calories: 553 | Carbs: 28g | Protein: 29.6g | Fat: 38.5g | Fiber: 9g

Ingredients:

- Two tbsps. of canola oil
- One cup each of
  - Onion (chopped)
  - Blended and shredded cheese (Mexican)
  - Chopped lettuce (romaine)
- One medium-sized tomato (diced)
- Two tsps. of cumin (ground)
- A quarter cup of prepared salsa (some extra for serving)
- One chopped avocado
- Three lb. of spaghetti squash, seeded and vertically sliced into halves
- Half a tsp. of salt
- Four tsps. of chili powder
- Three garlic (diced)
- One lb. of turkey (ground)

Method:

1. Set the oven at a temperature of 450 degrees F. Place a skillet over moderate flame and pour few oil drops. Then add the garlic, onion, and turkey. Cook for seven minutes, stirring occasionally and breaking the turkey chunks. Then add chili powder, salt, tomato, and cumin. Cook thoroughly for three minutes. Stir in the salsa after removing from heat.

2. Take a microwave-safe dish and place the cut-side down of squash on it. Add two tbsps. of water to the squash. Place the dish (uncovered) inside the microwave and bake for fifteen minutes. Make sure the squash flesh becomes tender.

3. Scrape out the flesh of squash from its shells with a fork. While the turkey mixture is still in the skillet, add the scooped squash flesh to it. Sprinkle remaining salt and then stir well.

4. Take a sheet (baking) and then arrange the squash shells on it. Scoop back the squash mixture into the shells. Top them with cheese. Thoroughly bake for fifteen minutes. Wait until the cheese melts and then top with avocado and lettuce. Serve with extra salsa if desired and enjoy.

Lemon Asparagus Chicken Skillet

Total Prep & Cooking Time: 35 minutes

Yields: Three plates

Nutrition Facts: Calories: 335 | Carbs: 14g | Protein: 36.9g | Fat: 15g | Fiber: 1.6g

Ingredients:

- Two tablespoons of avocado oil
- Half a teaspoon pepper
- One bunch of asparagus
- One-third cup of chicken broth
- One tablespoon of coconut aminos
- One teaspoon each of
  - Salt
  - Arrowroot starch
- One pound of chicken breast, sliced into cubes
- Three garlic cloves, minced
- One lemon juiced

Method:

1. Pour the avocado oil in the skillet and heat it over moderate heat.

2. After the oil starts to bubble out, add the chicken cubes and season with pepper and salt. Cook until the chicken becomes tender (insert the thermometer into the chicken's thickest part and check if it reads a

temperature of 165 degrees F) and then remove the chicken and set it aside.

3. To prepare the asparagus, chop off its thick white base and cut them vertically into halves.

4. Saute the asparagus for seven minutes with more pepper, oil, and salt if needed. They should become soft with a little crisp. Set them aside.

5. Lower the flame and then add the garlic to the skillet. Cook until it gives out the fragrance.

6. One by one, add the arrowroot starch, lemon juice, broth, and the coconut aminos. Stir them for about three minutes until the sauce attains a thickened consistency.

7. Add the asparagus and chicken pieces to the skillet and cook thoroughly for three more minutes.

8. Remove from the heat and top with onion wedges. Season more to satisfy your taste and finally serve it warm.

Note: This is an allergen-friendly meal that is made with foods that can provide you with the best of protein source and lime that is there to give a touch of acidic flavor. Chicken breast is good-to-go with this dish as it is easy to cook and makes things go smoother. You can omit the pepper part if you are on an AIP diet. Chicken broth is there to add the desired flavor and save the dish from getting thickened.

Egg Roll in a Bowl

Total Prep & Cooking Time: 30 minutes

Yields: Four servings

Nutrition Facts: Calories: 351 | Carbs: 15.8g | Protein: 38.2g | Fat: 15.8g | Fiber: 2.6g

Ingredients:

For preparing the roll,

- One pound of pork (ground)
- One diced onion (white)
- One teaspoon of ginger (grated)
- Two teaspoons of vinegar (apple cider)
- Two tablespoons each of
  - Chopped onion (green)
  - Sesame oil
- Two garlic cloves (diced)
- Twelve ounces of coleslaw mix
- Three tablespoons of coconut aminos

For preparing the sauce (optional),

- A quarter cup of coconut cream
- One teaspoon of vinegar (apple cider)

- Salt
- One tablespoon of coconut aminos
- Two teaspoons of freshly grated ginger

Method:

1. Take a large-sized skillet and cook the pork over moderate flame. Season with salt and pepper. Cook until the pork turns brown and then set it aside. You are recommended to dispose off the fat.

2. Pour some oil in the same skillet and heat over moderate flame. Once the oil starts to boil, add the ginger, garlic, and the onion to it. Cook to turn the onion translucent, and the garlic begins to give fragrance.

3. To the mixture, add the vinegar, coleslaw mix, and the coconut aminos— season with pepper and salt. Stir them properly for about five minutes.

4. Pour back the precooked pork to the skillet and then stir well. Saute the mixture for an additional minute.

5. Transfer the pork to the bowls. Top with the optional sauce and the onion. Serve and enjoy

For preparing the sauce,

1. Combine all ingredients for preparing the sauce and then stir well.

2. Serve the mixture over each bowl.

Note: *Coconut aminos is the substitute for the soy sauce. Avoid using a coleslaw mix that is too much filled with carrots to your dish extra sugary.*

One-pan Chicken Pesto

Total Prep & Cooking Time: 40 minutes

Yields: Three to Four plates of pesto

Nutrition Facts: Calories: 556 | Carbs: 24.5g | Protein: 43g | Fat: 32.5g | Fiber: 4.2g

Ingredients:

For preparing the sheet pan,

- Two pounds of chicken breast (you may substitute with chicken thigh), bone-in
- Two zucchinis (diced)
- One medium-sized red onion (finely chopped)
- Half a tsp. each of
  o Black pepper
  o Sea salt
- Two carrots (thinly sliced into circles)
- One sliced squash (yellow)

For preparing the mint basil pesto,

- One cup each of
  o Arugula
  o Basil (fresh)
- Two tablespoons of fresh mint
- A quarter cup of a freshly juiced lemon
- Half a tsp. of salt
- Half a cup of avocado oil
- One garlic clove (minced and peeled)

Method:

1. Add the ingredients for preparing the pesto into the blender and then process it. Do not turn the blender off until the mixture gets combined thoroughly. After you are done, set the mixture aside.

2. Set the oven at a temperature of 400 degrees F. you will require a baking sheet and a parchment paper. With the parchment paper, line the large-sized baking sheet.

3. Place all ingredients for preparing sheet pan on the sheet evenly. The ingredients must not be crowded. Coat the vegetables and the chicken properly with the pesto. Leave about two tablespoons of pesto for later use.

4. Place the baking sheet on the oven. After every ten minutes, flip the vegetables so that both sides are cooked evenly. Continue cooking for thirty-five minutes. After the said mark, insert a thermometer in the chicken's thickest part. If the reading shows 165 degrees F, then you may stop cooking. It means you have cooked the chicken thoroughly and have tenderized it.

5. Transfer the chicken to the plates. Top each plate with the leftover pesto and serve warm.

Note: An important part to note is that you should prevent overcrowding the pan in which you are cooking. The vegetables must be chopped with even thickness as it will ensure they finish cooking at the same time. The bone-in chicken is recommended as it leads to flavor enhancement and keeps the meat juicy.

BBQ Jackfruit

Total Prep & Cooking Time: 10 minutes

Yields: Two servings

Nutrition Facts: Calories: 471 | Carbs: 83.8g | Protein: 4.9g | Fat: 15.7g | Fiber: 4.7g

Ingredients:

- A can of jackfruit (fourteen ounces)
- Half a teaspoon of salt
- Two teaspoons each of
  - Onion powder
  - Garlic powder
  - Coconut sugar
- Two tablespoons each of
  - Avocado oil
  - Chopped green onion
- A quarter of black pepper
- One teaspoon of chili powder
- Half a cup of BBQ sauce

Method:

1. Remove the excess liquid from the jackfruit can.

2. Place a large-sized pan over a moderate flame. Then add jackfruit and sprinkle some salt, garlic, chili powder, coconut sugar, pepper, and onion. Stir well for three minutes until they soften.

3. Add the BBQ sauce to it and toss the veggies well to coat them with the sauce. Make the vegetables incorporated. Simmer for about three minutes.

4. Transfer the preparation to the plates. Top each plate with onions.

5. Serve warm and enjoy.

Chapter 4: How to Increase Immunity to Prevent Further Relapse?

If you're suffering from Hashimoto's, your thyroid gets inflamed because of the extra stress on your immune system, and as a result, the thyroid hormones are under-produced. You can prevent further relapses of Hashimoto disease and restore the optimal functions of your thyroid by increasing your immunity. You can boost your immunity and restore the function of your thyroid by using a few easy yet proven lifestyle and dietary changes (Premawardhana, 2006).

1. **Repair your gut** – It is essential to repair your gut if you have Hashimoto's. Almost eighty percent of your whole immune system is situated in your digestive system. The intestinal wall should be just a little permeable to allow the nutrients to reach the bloodstream. However, when it gets leaky, bigger molecules can enter your bloodstream and cause chronic inflammation. The immune system detects them as foreign invaders. Some of these invaders are very similar to the blood cells of the body, and so the immune system ends up attacking your thyroid accidentally. Thus, repairing the gut is extremely important. You can do it with the help of the amino acids and nutrients it requires and by eliminating inflammatory foods, parasites, infections, and toxins. You also need to re-inoculate with healthy bacteria and restore the acids and enzymes that are essential for proper digestion.

2. **Tame the toxins** – We are exposed to several hundreds of toxins in our daily lives. Toxins like nitrates, percolates, and mercury can accumulate in your body and impact your thyroid functions as they are chemically similar to iodine. You can, however, eliminate these toxins from your

body and prevent your exposure to them by taking a few necessary steps. Firstly, you need to learn how you are getting exposed to them and then try to minimize your exposure. After that, you can try detox pathways to flush the toxins safely from your body.

3. **Heal your infections** – Bacterial and viral infections can trigger Hashimoto's in various ways. Some common infections often don't show any symptoms. However, they can be tested for and treated.

4. **Relieve your stress** – Your adrenal gland produces and releases a large number of hormones when you're under stress. These signals make the stressor a priority and dismiss other functions, including the production of thyroid hormone and immune response. It can negatively affect your thyroid. Learning how to relieve stress can immensely help prevent the relapse of Hashimoto's. Walking, running, mediation, and deep breathing exercises can all help relieve stress and also prevent you from falling into a state of chronic stress.

PART II

Chapter 1: What in The World Is A Thyroid

In this chapter, we will be exploring just what the thyroid is, and its functions in maintaining and keeping your body healthy.

For starters, the word thyroid has its origins dating as far back as the 1690s. Coming from the Greek, *thyreoiedes,* meaning "shield-shaped". Also referred to as, *khondros thyreoiedes,* "shield-shaped cartilage". Aptly named, as the thyroid gland is an organ which is often considered to resemble a butterfly, bow tie, or shield shape, at the base of the neck.

The thyroid gland plays an extremely vital role in the way your body uses energy, by releasing hormones that aid in controlling your body's metabolism. The hormones released by the thyroid gland assist in regulating important body functions, including but not limited to:

- Regulation of breathing
- Heart rate
- The central and peripheral nervous systems
- Body weight
- Cycles of menstruation
- The strength of muscles
- Levels of cholesterol
- The temperature of the body

Quite a lot for an organ coming in at only around 2 inches long. This tiny but important gland rests in the front portion of the throat, in front of the trachea, and just below the thyroid cartilage commonly referred to as the Adam's apple. The Adam's apple itself is the largest cartilage of the voice box or larynx.

Owing to the bow tie, butterfly, or shield shape, of the thyroid gland, is a middle connection of thin thyroid tissue, which is known as the isthmus, which is responsible for holding together two lobes on the right and left sides of it. It is not entirely uncommon, however, for someone to be missing the isthmus all-together and instead of having the two lobes of the thyroid gland operating separate from one another.

Now that you are aware of this and may feel a bit more familiar with your own thyroid gland, you may resist trying to see or feel around for it in your neck yourself. Unless the thyroid gland is otherwise afflicted and made to become enlarged, mostly known as a goiter, the thyroid will be unable to be seen, and only just barely able to be felt. It is only when a goiter occurs and the neck is swollen from an enlarged thyroid that it will be at all noticeable either to the eye or to the touch.

The thyroid gland is one of the major players in the endocrine system. The endocrine system includes glands that are responsible for the production and for the secretion of various hormones. The other organs which help make up the endocrine system are the hypothalamus, which is responsible for linking the body's nervous system to the endocrine system via the use of the pituitary gland. The pituitary gland which is responsible for the secretion of hormones, not the blood stream. The pineal gland, which produces the wake/sleep pattern hormone of melatonin. The adrenal glands, which are responsible for the production of a variety of hormones like the steroids cortisol and aldosterone as well as our body's adrenaline. The Pancreas, an organ located in the abdominal region of the body, the primary role of which is the converting of food into fuel for the body's cells. The ovaries and testicles, sex organs of the body. And the parathyroid glands.

Utilizing the iodine content from foods, the thyroid is able to produce and churn out the hormones T3, which stands for triiodothyronine, and the hormone T4, thyroxine.

T3, or triiodothyronine, is merely the active form of the companion hormone thyroxine, or T4. The thyroid gland alone is able to secrete around 20% of our body's T3 into the bloodstream on its own. With the other 80% coming from organs like the liver and the kidneys going through the process of converting thyroxine into its active counterpart.

It is absolutely possible for your body to have far too much of T3 though. When there is an over secretion of T3 into the blood stream, it is called thyrotoxicosis. This can be due to a number of conditions dealing with the thyroid gland such as overactivity in the thyroid gland, known as hyperthyroidism, caused by such conditions as a benign tumor, the thyroid gland becoming enflamed, or a condition known as graves' disease. The previously mentioned condition of a goiter, in which the neck begins to swell, might be a signal of thyrotoxicosis having occurred. Even more symptoms to have an eye out for in case of hyperthyroidism will be an increase in the appetite, increased regularity of bowel movements, an intolerance to heat, the loss of weight, the menstrual cycle becoming irregulated, a heartbeat becoming increasingly rapid or irregular in rhythm, the thinning or loss of hair, tremors, becoming irritable, overly tired, palpitations, and the eyelids retracting.

It is also possible for your body to be producing too little of the hormone T3. The thyroid gland producing too little of T3 is known commonly as hypothyroidism. It is common for autoimmune diseases to have a strong role in this occurring, an example of which would be the Hashimoto's disease, which causes the immune system to attack the thyroid gland. Certain medications or the intake of too little iodine can also cause hypothyroidism. This can be very serious, especially if a case of hypothyroidism goes unnoticed or untreated during early childhood, or even before birth. With the regulation of hormones being so important, primarily to physical and mental development, not treating hypothyroidism during these crucial times often result in reduced growth for the child, or becoming learning disabled.

The affliction of hypothyroidism is not foreign to adults though. When hypothyroidism occurs in adults they tend to have the functions of their bodies slowed down drastically. The effects of hypothyroidism in an adult have been known to include symptoms such as a growing intolerance to colder temperature, the heart rate of the adult will lower, gaining weight, a reduction in appetite, the ability of memory becomes poorer, fertility will reduce, muscles will become stiff, the adult may become depressed, and tired.

T4, or thyroxine, is the primary hormone that gets secreted from the thyroid gland and into the body's bloodstream. Unlike T3 which is active, thyroxine is in an inactive form and most of it will need to be converted to the active form, triiodothyronine, which is a process that takes place in organs like the kidneys and liver. Undergoing these processes is vital in making sure the body is able to regulate a healthy metabolic rate, control of the body's muscles, development of the brain, develop and maintain bones, and digestive and heart functionality.

As with T3, triiodothyronine, the production and secretion of too much will inevitable result in thyrotoxicosis, while the production and secretion of too little thyroxine, will result in hypothyroidism.

To combat this, the body and thyroid gland have a few tricks vital to the regulation of levels of these hormones in the cells. There is a controlled feedback loop system, involving the hypothalamus in the brain as well as in the thyroid gland and pituitary gland which is in control of the production of both of the hormones thyroxine and triiodothyronine. Thyrotropin-releasing hormones are secreted from the hypothalamus and, in turn, the pituitary gland becomes stimulated into producing thyroid stimulating hormone. A hormone which will stimulate thyroxine and triiodothyronine to be produced and secreted by the thyroid gland.

A feedback loop regulates this production system, to account for the levels of thyroxine and of triiodothyronine. If the levels of either of these thyroid gland hormones begin to increase, they will end up preventing the production and secretion of the thyrotropin-releasing hormone as well as the thyroid stimulating hormone, thus allowing the body to maintain, on it's own, a steady level of the thyroid hormones that it needs.

For all these reasons it is of vital importance that the levels of T3 and T4 being secreted thru-ought the body and its cells never get too high or too low. T3 and T4 are able to reach just about ever cell in the body by utilizing the bloodstream. The rate of work for the cells and metabolism to work is regulated by the hormones T3 and T4. To make sure that levels are never either too high or too low, this is why we have a thyroid gland.

The final hormone that the thyroid gland is responsible for the production of is the hormone calcitonin, CT, or thyrocalcitonin. Within the thyroid gland are what are known as C-cells, or parafollicular cells, which are in charge of the proliferation of this particular hormone. The primary role of calcitonin in the body is to help in the regulation of the levels of phosphate in the blood, and of calcium in the blood. Doing so is to be in opposition of the parathyroid hormone. In short, meaning that what it aims to do is reduce the amount of calcium in the blood stream. The reason for playing this role in the human anatomy game has been a bit of a mystery to science up to this point though, due to the observation of patients showing either very high or even very low levels of the hormone calcitonin, having no adverse effect on them.

The hormone calcitonin has two primary mechanisms by which to aid in the reduction of calcium levels within the human body. It can completely inhibit the activity of the cells in our body which are responsible for breaking down bones, known as osteoclasts. Osteoclasts do this because when bone is broken down, the calcium within the bone being broken down will be released into the body's bloodstream. So by inhibiting the osteoclasts from doing their respective jobs, calcitonin is directly involved in the reduction of the amount of calcium that is getting released into the body's bloodstream. Despite doing this though, the length of time that calcitonin can cause this inhibition has been shown to be quite short. Calcitonin can be an active player in the resorption of calcium into the kidneys, which it does by lower the levels of blood calcium in the body.

Calcitonin has been manufactured in the past and has then been given, in this form, to treat the disease of bone, Paget's disease. Also known as osteitis deformans, Paget's disease is rather common, and is a chronic bone disorder which can cause pain, fractures or deformities of a bone, or show absolutely no symptoms at all. It is however easily able to be controlled and treated with proper early enough diagnosis and treatment.

The manufactured hormone calcitonin has also been given to sufferers of general bone pain, and of hypercalcaemia, which is when the body has an abnormal level of calcium flowing in the bloodstream.

Though because of the introduction of bisphosphonates, which aid in the preventing of the breakdown of bone cells and are drugs also used to help treat osteoporosis, the use of manufactured calcitonin has decreased.

Chapter 2: Possible Thyroid Disorders

In the previous chapter, we began to cover what it is exactly that the thyroid gland gets done and even dabbled a bit into how it does it's job properly. During the last chapter, we mentioned a few of the various thigs which can afflict the thyroid gland, why this may occur in certain circumstances, and what the effects of these afflictions could be. Moving on into chapter two is where we will begin to take a closer look at everything that can go wrong with the thyroid gland. Not just the what, but the why as well. What causes these changes in our thyroid gland to occur, and what to expect to happen when they do occur. The importance of having this knowledge be a part of your thyroid gland arsenal cannot be at all overstated as there is a wide array of severity to both the symptoms and to the results of the ailments that can afflict the thyroid gland and consequently hinder our body's ability to maintain its health properly.

Just as well in this chapter, you can expect to be reading deeper into some of the ailments that may have already been brought up in the previous chapter, such as hyperthyroidism, hypothyroidism, graves disease, goiters, and Hashimoto's disease.

Hyperthyroidism

As briefly discussed in the last chapter, hyperthyroidism is a rather common condition in which there is overactivity in the thyroid gland and begins to produce far too much of the thyroid hormone which would usually be used to regulate the body's metabolic rate. This can be an overproduction of the hormones T3, which is triiodothyronine, T4, which is tetraiodothyronine, or even an overproduction of both of these hormones.

The causes of hyperthyroidism can vary greatly, with the most common reason for it being the aforementioned Grave's disease, which we will go much further into later in the chapter. The basics of Grave's disease are that it is an autoimmune disorder which causes antibodies in the body to stimulate the thyroid gland making it secrete to many of it's hormones. You should tell your regular doctor if any one in your family has ever had Grave's disease as it seems to have a genetic link, being passed down commonly from generation to the next generation. Grave's disease is also known to be more prevalent in women, affecting about 1 percent of the female population, than it is in men.

Another common reason for hyperthyroidism to occur is an excess level of iodine in the body, which is the main ingredient in hormones T3 and T4.

Less common, but still just as relevant to the conversation as causes for hyperthyroidism is thyroiditis which is the inflammation of thyroid gland, which in turn will cause the hormones T3 and T4 to start leaking out of the thyroid gland.

Tumors located on the ovaries or testes have been known links to hyperthyroidism. As well as even tumors, even when benign, located on the thyroid gland, or pituitary gland.

An easily preventable cause of hyperthyroidism which should not be overlooked is the intake of large amounts of T4, or tetraiodothyronine, via the ingestion of a dietary supplement or of a prescribed medication.

When it comes to the symptoms of hyperthyroidism, believe it or not, we had only scratched the surface in the previous chapter and will be going more in-depth here on what you can expect to look out for in order to self-diagnose an issue before going to seek out a professional opinion.

To begin with, in the case of Grave's disease, one of the symptoms can be a bulging of the eyes as if stuck in a stare. Other symptoms to watch out for would be an increase in the appetite, perhaps an increase in nervousness or a sense of restlessness. Muscular weakness, the inability to concentrate on simple tasks, irregularity in the heartbeat, loss of the ability to sleep soundly or for long periods of time, the loss of hair, or noticing that your hair has become thinner or more brittle, can be signs of hyperthyroidism. Thinness of the skin is also common, as well as becoming more irritable, sweating more, or becoming more anxious. In men specifically, the development of breasts can be a sign of hyperthyroidism. And in women, hyperthyroidism has been known to have adverse effects on the regularity of the menstrual cycle.

If you experience any of the prior symptoms, it is, of course, recommended to seek out professional help and diagnosis. However, it is highly recommended that you seek out professional help for the treatment of hyperthyroidism if you begin to experience a sensation of dizziness if you start to notice shortness in your breathing, which will likely come with the increase in heart rate, making it faster and irregular, and any loss of consciousness. Having hyperthyroidism has also been known to be the cause of atrial fibrillations, which are a dangerous arrythmia, commonly responsible for leading to having a stroke, or even to congestive heart failures.

In diagnosing a case of hyperthyroidism, a doctor will likely begin the process by conducting a full and complete medical history, as well as a physical exam. These are commonly conducted as they are helpful in revealing the common signs of loss of weight, how rapid your pulse is, an elevation in pressure of the blood, protrusion of the eyes, or the enlargement of the thyroid gland itself.

It is also reasonable to expect your doctor to conduct a cholesterol test which will be done to check on the levels of cholesterol in your system. This is done because cholesterol levels being low can be an indication that there is an elevation in your metabolic rate, which would mean that your body is burning through your cholesterol far too quickly.

Doctors are also able to conduct tests to measure the levels of T3 and T4 that are in your blood. Thyroid stimulating hormone tests can be done to check the levels of TSH, or thyroid stimulating hormone coursing within your body. TSH stimulates your thyroid gland to produce the hormones the body needs, and if your thyroid gland is producing levels of hormones at a normal rate, or even a rate that is too high, your TSH should come out lower. And a level of TSH that is abnormally low can be an important signifier that you may have hyperthyroidism.

A triglyceride test will be done, because similarly to having low amounts of cholesterol, a low level of triglycerides can be significant of an elevation in your metabolic rate. A thyroid scan or uptake will allow a doctor to see if your thyroid gland is being overactive. It will actually get even more particular, and let a doctor be able to see if it is the entire thyroid gland which is acting up or just a particular area of the thyroid gland.

Ultrasounds have been known to be utilized, as they will allow a doctor to observe entirely, the size of the thyroid gland, as well as any masses that may be within the thyroid gland. It is the use of the ultrasound which will also be able to let the doctor know if the mass inside the thyroid gland is cystic, or if it is solid. Just as well a CT, Computed Tomography, or MRI, Magnetic Resonance Imaging, scan can be performed to show if the condition is being caused by a tumor being present on the pituitary gland.

Treatment of hyperthyroidism also comes in varieties and may be dependent on the cause of the hyperthyroidism. Perhaps the most common treatment comes in the form of medication. Generally an antithyroid medication like methimazole, also known as Tapazole, which will cause the thyroid gland to halt the production and secretion of hormones altogether.

According to the American Thyroid Association, around 70 percent of U.S. adults who undergo treatment for hyperthyroidism will receive a form of treatment called radioactive iodine. Radioactive iodine is essentially able to completely and effectively destroy the cells that would otherwise be producing hormones. Radioactive iodine, or RAI, in the form of a liquid or a pill, will be ingested by way of the mouth, and is safe to use on an individual who has had any allergic reaction to an X-ray contrast agent or to seafood, because essentially the reaction comes from the compound which contains iodine, and not from the iodine itself. The iodine, in an iodide form, is actually split into two forms or radioactive iodine, known as I-123, which is harmless to thyroid gland cells, and I-131, which is responsible for the destruction of thyroid gland cells. The radiation which is emitted by both of these forms of the iodine are able to be detected from outside of the patient, which will help the doctor to gain any information needed the thyroid glands functionality, and take any pictures needed of the size thyroid glands tissues, as well as their location in the body. This treatment is not without its side effects though, which generally tend to come in the presence of dryness of the mouth, soreness of the eyes and in the throat, and has also been known to effect changes in taste. You may also be required, if undergoing this treatment, to take precautions for a short time which will prevent the spread of radiation to others.

Surgery is yet another common form of treatment for hyperthyroidism. In this case, it is entirely possible that a section of your thyroid gland will be removed, though entire thyroid glands have also been removed in this procedure. This is followed up with taking thyroid hormone supplements which will help in the prevention of hypothyroidism, which is what happens when there is the occurrence of underactivity in the thyroid gland, causing it to produce and secrete too little of the intended hormones. Beta-blockers may also be taken, such as something like propranolol to help control a rapid pulse, sweating, any anxiety that may crop up, and higher blood pressure. It is reported that most people respond very well to this form of treatment.

If you would like to improve any symptoms, or even take action to prevent symptoms from occurring, you are not left without options. You can work along with your doctor, or a dietician, to help create a healthy guideline for diet, exercise, and any nutritional supplementation. Proper diet intake, with a stronger focus on getting calcium and sodium, can be crucially important in the prevention of hyperthyroidism. Osteoporosis is a common result of hyperthyroidism as it can make your bones become thin, weak, and very brittle. To strengthen the bones after treatment for hyperthyroidism, it is recommended to take calcium supplements and vitamin D. To get an idea of how much vitamin D you should be taking post-surgery, you can talk to your doctor for a recommendation.

Moving on from treatment, it is not unusual for a doctor to recommend their patients to an endocrinologist, who will be more specialized in the treatment of systems dealing with bodily hormones. You'll want to avoid stress at this stage as it can cause thyroid storm, which happens when a large amount of thyroid hormone gets released, resulting in a horrible and sudden worsening of any prior symptoms. Proper treatment is both recommended and effective at the prevention of thyroid storm, as well as other complications such as thyrotoxicosis.

In the long-term, the outlook for something like hyperthyroidism is dependent heavily on what is causing it. Some of the causes of hyperthyroidism can go away without ever seeking treatment. Whereas a more serious cause like Graves' disease is not to be taken lightly, as it will get much worse if it goes without treatment, and the complications due to Graves' disease are often life-threatening and will have an affect on your quality of life long-term. These are easy enough to subdue with proper care and an early diagnosis and treatment.

Hypothyroidism

Though we went over a little about hypothyroidism in chapter 1, it is important to take a closer look at the disorder, to gain a better idea of its symptoms, and proper treatment and care for it.

When the body is not producing enough of the thyroid hormones that it needs, this is what is known as hypothyroidism having occurred. This will cause the general functions of your body to become slowed down, as the thyroid gland is responsible for producing and secreting hormones which will provide energy to nearly every other portion of your body. Though this affliction can come to task at any age, it is more common for an underactive thyroid gland to be noticed in adults over the age of 60, as well as being more prevalent in women. A diagnosis of hypothyroidism is nothing to get too worked up about, fortunately, as treatment of hypothyroidism has been known to be quite effective, as well as being very simple and very safe.

Though the symptoms of having an underactive thyroid gland can vary from person to person, there is enough overlap in the symptoms for us to help lay out what to look out for. It is important to note, however, that there can be difficulty in pin-pointing that a symptom is that of hypothyroidism and that the severity of the condition itself plays a large role in which signs or symptoms will appear, as well as when they may make an appearance.

It is not at all uncommon for most people to experience the symptoms of this condition arriving in a slow progression over many years. The thyroid gland will grow ever slower and slower, which will only then allow the symptoms to be better identifiable. The trouble can become that many of the symptoms come with general aging, so if you suspect there is more to the picture, and that hypothyroidism is at play, it is important to go see a doctor. An example of some early symptoms which also come naturally with age are the symptomatic fatigue and gaining of weight.

If hypothyroidism does occur, however, other symptoms to keep an eye out for will be an uptick in depression, constipation, or muscle weakness. It is also common to begin becoming more sensitive to the cold, for the skin to become dry, and a reduction in sweating. Your heart rate will generally become slower, blood cholesterol may elevate, and joints may become stiff or experience more pain. It is also possible for memory to start becoming impaired, hair may thin or become dry. Your voice may become hoarse, muscles will stiffen and experience soreness, your face will become puffy and sensitive. In women, hypothyroidism as been known to negatively affect menstrual changes and cause difficulty in fertility.

When it comes to the causes of hypothyroidism, an autoimmune disease is fairly common to be the culprit at work. The body is designed in such a way that your immune system generally will protect the body's cells against any invading bacteria and virus. Therefore, when an unknown virus or bacteria enters the body, it is the immune system which will respond by sending out what are known as fighter cells, to destroy the foreign invading virus or bacteria.

However, it is not impossible for your body to begin confusing what are the healthy and normal cells, with the invading cells. This is what is then called an autoimmune response to the cells. And if this autoimmune response does not get properly treated, or if it is not properly regulated, it is your own immune system which will start to attack your healthy body tissues. Medically, this has been known to cause quite serious issues, which include hypothyroidism.

Hashimoto's disease, which we have mentioned before, is one such autoimmune condition that can occur, and it is the most common among the causes of having an underactive thyroid gland. The disease literally will attack the thyroid gland which will cause chronic thyroid inflammation, which, in turn, will reduce the functionality of the thyroid gland. As with Graves' disorder having links between generations, it is not at all uncommon to find that multiple members of a family have this same condition as well.

Hypothyroidism can even become an occurrence as a result of treatment for hyperthyroidism, which has the aim of lowering your thyroid hormone. It is not uncommon for the treatment to result in keeping the thyroid hormone too low, which then becomes hypothyroidism, which has been a known result of the radioactive iodine treatment for hyperthyroidism.

The surgical removal of the thyroid gland is yet another known cause of the occurrence of hypothyroidism. The entirety of the thyroid gland will be removed in the case of thyroid problems cropping up, which will affect the body's ability to produce thyroid hormone, and cause hypothyroidism. In this instance, you will typically be recommended to take thyroid medication for the rest of your life. In the case that it is only a smaller portion of the thyroid gland which is removed, it is possible for the thyroid gland to still be able to produce and secrete a healthy amount of hormones. In which case it will take a test of the blood to determine how much medication you will need.

It is possible for radiation therapy to be the cause if you have come down with hypothyroidism. A diagnosis of leukemia, neck cancer, or lymphoma will likely mean you have had to undergo a form of radiation therapy, which very nearly almost leads to the occurrence of hypothyroidism.

Just as possible, is a medication you may be taking to lower thyroid gland hormone production, to be the cause of hypothyroidism. Medications such as these are commonly used in the treatment of certain psychological diseases, and even have been known to be used in treating heart disease and cancer.

When it comes down the diagnosing of hypothyroidism, there are two primary methods which have been favored and work to best identify when it has occurred. The first being a strict medical evaluation, much like in the case of checking for hyperthyroidism. The doctor will give you a very thorough exam physically, as well as making sure to go over your medical history. Hypothyroidism has a couple physical signs which the doctor will be checking for primarily such as the dryness of the skin, how slow or quick your reflexes are, any swelling of the neck, and the rate of your heart beat. It is at this time that a doctor will also likely ask you to report any of the other symptoms listed earlier that you may have experienced, such as the depression, any fatigue, if you have been constipated, and a sensation of being more sensitive to the cold. It is also at this point it will be most helpful for you to let the doctor know of any thyroid conditions which have existed in your family.

To reliably get an idea of the existence of hypothyroidism in the body, it is required to conduct blood tests. It is only by this method that anyone will be able to tell and get a look at a measure of your body's thyroid-stimulating hormone levels, done by utilizing a thyroid-stimulating hormone test to see how much of the thyroid-stimulating hormone your pituitary gland is or is not creating. In the case that your thyroid gland is not producing enough of the hormone, the pituitary gland will respond to this by boosting the thyroid-stimulating hormone it produces in order to increase thyroid hormone production. If it turns out you have hypothyroidism, the levels of thyroid-stimulating hormone in your body will be increased, because your body is responding by making an attempt at stimulating more thyroid gland hormone activity. If hyperthyroidism is what ails you, the levels of the thyroid-stimulating hormone in your body will as having decreased, because in this case, your body has begun the process of attempting to halt the function of excessive production of the thyroid glands hormones.

Another useful method in the detection and diagnosis of hypothyroidism is to test the levels of T4 in the body, being produced by your thyroid gland, as T4 is produced directly by the thyroid gland. When they are used in conjunction with one another, a test of T4 levels and the thyroid-stimulating hormone test are very helpful in coming up with an evaluation of thyroid gland functionality. In general, if you the levels of thyroid-stimulating hormone in your body has increased, while the level of the hormone T4 has decreased, you much more than likely have hypothyroidism. Though, due to the sheer amount of conditions that can have such a negative impact on the thyroid gland, it could very well end up being necessary to conduct even more tests of the thyroid glands function I order to properly diagnose the issue.

Though it is true that for many people who have thyroid conditions, that the right amount of the proper medication will assist in the alleviation of their symptoms, you will have hypothyroidism for the rest of your life if you get it.

To get the best of hypothyroidism it is most commonly treated the best with the use of levothyroxine, also known as Levothroid or Levoxyl, which is T4 put into a synthetic form that is responsible for copying the action the thyroid hormone would regularly take if it were being produced as normal by your body. The idea behind doing this is that the medication will cause a return to the proper levels of the thyroid hormone in your blood. Once a restoration of the thyroid hormone level has occurred, many of the symptoms that come along with having hypothyroidism, will at the very least become much easier to manage, and at best the hypothyroidism symptoms will disappear altogether. It is important to expect it to take several weeks, following treatment, before relief sets in, and you start to feel a return to normalcy. There will also very likely be follow up appointments for testing your blood, which the doctor will recommend in order to keep a solid eye on your progress into recovery. Chances are that you will also receive some medication or other recommended methods to aid you in your recovery, be sure to speak with your doctor about the dosage you should be taking and to come up with a solid plan, that will most benefit you, for recovering in a timely fashion.

It is the case that many people who end up with hypothyroidism medicate for it, for the rest of their lives. Despite this, the dosage you will be taking thru ought that time is likely to go through changes. To better get an idea of how these dosages should be changing over time, it is best to get a check up on your thyroid-stimulation hormone levels every year. In this way, your doctor will be able to more properly adjust the amount you should be taking, or not taking, based on the blood levels indicated by the thyroid-stimulating hormone tests. Only by doing this regularly, will you and your doctor be able to achieve the recovery program that works best for you.

Plans and programs for this achievement may include medications and other hormone supplementation. Once again, synthetic versions of the hormone you need may be used, as they are a widely used and viable practice to aid in the recovery of hypothyroidism. The synthetic version of the hormone T3 is liothyronine, and T4 in its synthetic medication form is called levothyroxine, both of which act as suitable substitutes for their corresponding hormone.

If it was a deficiency in your iodine intake which caused your specific occurrence of hypothyroidism, it is likely that your doctor will recommend a supplementary form of iodine. Keep in mind to ask your doctor, and get the proper testing before taking anything, but selenium and magnesium supplements have been known to aid heavily in the treatment of hypothyroidism.

The golden ticket to any recovery or treatment is usually diet, and in the case of hypothyroidism, there is no exception. Though this is the case, and diet can be incredibly beneficial in your recovery and treatment, do not expect a change in your diet, doctor recommended or otherwise, to replace the need for a prescribed medication. Foods that are rich in selenium or magnesium such as nuts and seeds like the Brazil nut and sunflower seeds have been shown to be very beneficial additions to any diet to aid in the treatment of hypothyroidism.

Balance in your diet will play an especially important role, as the thyroid gland requires particular amounts of iodine in order to properly reach full functionality. There are foods such as whole grains, vegetables, fruits, and lean meats which can handily accomplish this without the need for iodine supplementation.

And of course, diet is only the beginning, exercise as well comes in as an important slice of the treatment and recovery pie. The muscle and joint pain that coincides with hypothyroidism will more often than not leave one to feel extreme fatigue and depression, both of which can be helped by creating and sticking to a regular work out regime. Though no exercise should be discounted, unless specifically told to avoid certain activities by your doctor, there are certain ones which will prove more beneficial than others for treating the symptoms of hypothyroidism. Low impact workouts such as swimming, riding a bike, doing Pilates or yoga, or even a good brisk walk, have been known to be very helpful low impact work outs that are helpful and easy to work in to a daily routine.

The building up of muscle mass by strength training, lifting weights, sit ups, pushups, and pull-ups, help reduce the lethargic feeling of sluggishness that comes along with hypothyroidism. The increase in muscle mass will result in an increase in the rate of your metabolism, which will simultaneously assist in decreasing any weight gain that the hypothyroidism may have caused.

And finally doing training that is primarily cardiovascular. As stated earlier, hypothyroidism is one of the ailments that can correlate with a heightened risk of having a cardiac arrythmia, or irregularity of the heartbeat. By taking steps to be more mindful of your cardiovascular health, exercising on a regular basis or schedule, will help in protecting your heart.

There are also alternative treatments which exist to help in taking care of hypothyroidism, such as animal extracts that contain the thyroid hormone. These extracts are made available from pigs because they contain both the thyroid hormone T4 and thyroid hormone T3. It is uncommon for these to be recommended, however, as they have not shown to be reliable in how to dose, as well as not being more effective than the typically recommended medications. It is also popular to find some glandular extracts in stores that are health food based. The risk that comes along with them is that the U.S. Food and Drug Administration plays no role in the monitoring or the regulation of these extracts. This has historically brought the guarantee of their pureness, legitimacy, and even their potency into question. If you decide to use these products, you do so at your own risk, but still be sure to inform your doctor so that they can adjust accordingly to your treatment.

You can go above and beyond in regards to hypothyroidism treatment, yet still deal with issues or complications that are longer lasting because of this harsh fluctuation to your body. Luckily there have been methods developed and used which will help to lessen the burden of hypothyroidisms effects on your life moving forward.

In the beginning, fatigue can feel like a lot to deal with, especially when associated with depression. These feelings can creep through even if you are taking proper dosages of your medication. It is of utmost importance that you get a good quality sleep every night to ease your treatment and recovery. A good, healthy diet, as well as the relief of stress through activities such as meditation, Pilates, and yoga, are effective strategies when it comes to combating lower energy levels.

It is also vitally important to recognize the difficulty of having a medical condition that is chronic, especially in the case of something like hypothyroidism, which comes along with its own mixed bag of other concerns to your overall health. Being able to talk about, or express, the experience of going through this will help. There are resources out there for support groups of other people who live with the effects of hypothyroidism, you can find a therapist to talk to, perhaps a close friend or loved one. Anyone who will be able to enable you to discuss your experience with openness and with honesty. You may even be able to receive a recommendation for meetings of people with hypothyroidism, from an education office at your local hospital. Connecting and communicating with others who can empathize with what you are going through could end up being an enormous aid in your recovery and life with hypothyroidism.

Important as well is making sure you monitor yourself for other health conditions that could arise. As we went over earlier, the main cause for hypothyroidism is an autoimmune disease. Just as well, links with hypothyroidism have also been found in conditions such as diabetes, having pituitary issues, having your sleep obstructed by sleep apnea, and lupus.

Just as with fatigue, depression is a common symptom and side effect of going through and living with hypothyroidism and should be watched closely. The thyroid glands hormone levels lower, the function of your body begins to slow down, and before you may realize it you are living with a depression that was not there before. It is vital to know what to look out for, and not just what, but also how to look after yourself while dealing with this.

Depression as a symptom can make hypothyroidism difficult to diagnose as there are many who may only experience difficulties or changes in mood as a symptom. It is for this reason, that instead of having a doctor check only your brain when checking for depression, it can also be important to ask them to check for signs of you having an underactive thyroid. Aside from the changes in mood, there are a few other similarities that exist in both having depression as well as hypothyroidism such as, gaining weight, finding it difficult to maintain concentration, feelings of daily fatigue, which coincide with a reduced desire and satisfaction with daily life, and hypothyroidism or depression could both effect your ability to sleep well.

Not all of their symptoms overlap so nicely though, both have their conditions which differentiate one from the other. In the case of hypothyroidism there are, of course, some physical signs such as the dryness of the skin, or the thinning and loss of hair. There is also the tendency to become constipated and the increase in levels of cholesterol.

These symptoms would be atypical if depression alone was the issue.

If you have hypothyroidism and it is the cause of your depression, then the correct treatment and care of the hypothyroidism should be just the remedy needed in order to treat your depression as well. If the hypothyroidism passes and depression remains, it may be important to talk to your doctor about receiving further help and a change in medication.

Along with depression being a symptom of hypothyroidism, it has recently been found, through studies, that around 60 percent or so of people who get hypothyroidism tend to also exhibit having anxiety as well. Studies are ongoing and are still growing in scope and size, though it would still be in your best interest to discuss all possibilities and symptoms with your doctor in order to more thoroughly and best tackle the treatment of hypothyroidism.

It cannot be stressed enough, how much of your body is under the affects and influence of your thyroid gland working properly to produce and secrete the correct levels of hormones. For this reason, when a woman gets hypothyroidism and simultaneously desires to get pregnant, she will be faced with her own subset of challenges to come. Have a low thyroid gland function during a pregnancy can cause a number of conflicts including various birth defects, have a still-birth or miscarriage, as well as anemia or a low birth weight. It is not uncommon for a woman with thyroid problems to have a perfectly healthy pregnancy, but to make sure that you reach this outcome it is important to do things such as eating well, keeping yourself informed about current and effective medicines, as well as talking to your doctor about testing.

Though testing may result in changes to your dosage or medication, it is also for this reason that it is important to make sure you are not deviating from the medications provided and the dosage your doctor has recommended.

Considering the thyroid issues adds on even more importance to the need for eating healthy while pregnant. Make sure that you are getting the proper amount of vitamins, minerals, and nutrients and consider taking multivitamins as well to supplement this.

It is not impossible to develop a thyroid issue such as hypothyroidism while pregnant. In fact, for every 1,000 pregnancies, this tends to occur in every 3 out of 5 women. It is important for doctors to routinely check thyroid levels during your pregnancy, as some will do, to make sure your thyroid levels aren't becoming to high or low. If they end up being higher or lower than they ought to be, it is likely that your doctor will recommend you starting treatment. Even some women who have never before had any thyroid issues may develop them once the baby is born, which is known as postpartum thyroiditis, and also tends to resolve itself after a year in around 80 percent of the women it shows up in. It is only the other 20 percent of women who will have this happen and then go on to require the long term treatment.

When hypothyroidism takes place, and the functions of the body slow down, it is quite typical for people to become prone to gaining weight, which is very likely due to what happens to the bodies ability to burn energy, which is that the efficiency to do so slows down as well. This change in the body will typically cause someone who has hypothyroidism to gain anywhere from 5 to 10 pounds in general, making the weight that is gained not entirely drastic, but someone could still find it quite alarming. It is very possible then, that once the hypothyroidism has been treated, that any weight gained will then be easily lost. If this does not occur, a simple change in diet, and adding regular exercise to your routine should aid in handily losing the weight, as your ability to manage weight will go back to normalcy, with the return to proper levels in your thyroid hormones.

Hypothyroidism is a common occurrence; therefore it is also commonly treated without issue. Hypothyroidism has been found to occur in around 4.6 percent of the American population that are 12 and older. Which comes out to about 10 million or so people who go on to live long healthy lives with the condition, and you may never even realize it. It is far more prevalent in people who are over the age of 60, and in women about 1 in 5 of them are likely to experience hypothyroidism by the time they have reached 60 years of age. One of the causes is Hashimoto's disease which happens to appear more in women who have reached middle-age, though it can absolutely show up in children and men. As Hashimoto's disease is hereditary, it is likely that if you get it, you did so from a relative, and have an increased chance then of passing it on down to your children.

It is important to keep an eye on your body, your health, and your thyroid gland as you get older. If, as the years go by, you begin to notice any of the changes gone over in this chapter so far, it is vital that you see a doctor in an attempt to get a proper diagnosis and seek treatment as soon as possible.

Hashimoto's Disease

Hashimoto's disease is an autoimmune disease which can be very destructive to your thyroid gland, and thereby your thyroid glands ability to function properly. Hashimoto's disease is also known as chronic autoimmune lymphocytic thyroiditis and is the most common cause of having an underactive thyroid gland, hypothyroidism, in the United States.

As an autoimmune disorder, Hashimoto's disease is one of many conditions that will be the cause of your body's white blood cells and your body's antibodies becoming confused and starting to attack the cells that make up the thyroid gland. What makes this happen precisely is still somewhat of a mystery to doctors, even still it is believed by some that factors of genetics may be involved.

With the cause of Hashimoto's disease being unknown, it is difficult to precisely put a finger on what puts a person at risk for having or contracting the disease. There are still, however, just a few factors that doctors are aware of which could signify being at risk for the disease. In the case of Hashimoto's disease, in particular, women happen to be seven times more likely to contract than men, and especially for women who have been pregnant before. Having a history of autoimmune diseases in the family is another factor that could mean you are at higher risk of having Hashimoto's at some point in your life, especially if the autoimmune diseases include Graves' disease, lupus, rheumatoid arthritis, if there is a history of Sjogren's syndrome in your family, or a history of type 1 diabetes, Addison's disease, and vitiligo. If it is the case that these autoimmune diseases are present in your family line or may have been based on symptoms of Hashimoto's disease, get together and discuss the possibility with your doctor, then make sure to get tested for the disease.

Hashimoto's disease is interesting in that the symptoms of it, are not symptomatic of Hashimoto's disease alone, in fact, they are similar to having the symptoms of an underactive thyroid gland, or hypothyroidism. Some signs to watch out for that your thyroid gland is not working properly to produce proper thyroid hormones, and that you may have Hashimoto's disease are your skin becoming dry and pale, constipation, if your voice becomes hoarse, you become depressed and start to feel sluggish or fatigued. High levels of cholesterol, a thinning of the hair, muscle weakness in the lower body, and intolerance to the cold may also be signs of hypothyroidism as a result of Hashimoto's disease. In women, it can also cause issues with fertility. Hashimoto's can exist inside of your body for many years before you begin to show any signs or symptoms, and during that time, it may progress while showing no signs of damage to the thyroid gland. Some with Hashimoto's disease end up with a goiter, an enlarging of the thyroid gland which causes the front of the neck to swell. Though generally painless, it is common for a goiter to make the act of swallowing difficult and for it to simulate a feeling of fullness in the throat.

Owing to it's difficulty to diagnose, your doctor may not suspect Hashimoto's of being prevalent until observing symptoms having hypothyroidism. In which case they will need to conduct a blood test designed to check the thyroid-stimulating hormone, or TSH, levels in your body. It is a relatively common and safe test, which is also an accurate way to check to see if you have Hashimoto's disease. Levels of thyroid-stimulating hormone are higher when the activity of the thyroid glad is lower because your body starts working harder to stimulate the production of more thyroid hormones to secrete from the thyroid gland. There are also blood tests that your doctor may conduct if they feel the need to check further for the levels of antibodies, cholesterol, and other thyroid hormones, T3 and T4, in your blood. Testing for all of these can help immensely in pinning down a diagnosis of Hashimoto's disease.

Unless your thyroid gland is functioning normally, in which case your doctor may still recommend regular checkups to monitor you for any changes, it is very likely that the need for treatment of Hashimoto's disease will be required.

The improper production of enough hormones in your body by your thyroid gland will likely result in the need to take medication. In the case of having to take this medication, it is also likely that you will be prescribed on it, though dose will vary, for the rest of your life. The effective drug most commonly prescribed is levothyroxine which is the hormone thyroxine, or T4, made synthetically, and which will successfully replace the missing hormone in your blood. The synthetic hormone drug levothyroxine tends not to have any noticeable side effects, and regular use has been known to frequently return the hormone levels of the body back to normal, restoring proper function of the thyroid gland. When this happens, all other symptoms of Hashimoto's disease and hypothyroidism generally tend to disappear altogether, though it is likely that your doctor will still recommend that you still get regular testing done so that your hormone levels can be consistently monitored to prevent something like hypothyroidism from becoming a problem again moving forward. Getting the regular testing allows the doctor to adjust the dosage of your medication as necessary if at all necessary.

It is important to consider before going on levothyroxine, that there are supplements and medications which will have an effect on your body's ability to absorb the drug. As such, make sure you have a discussion about this with your doctor if you are taking any other medications, especially if they include iron or calcium supplements, or estrogen. Some medications for cholesterol have been known to cause an issue, as well as proton pump inhibitors which are used as a treatment for acid reflux.

Though these have been known to cause an issue, there is what could be an easy work around of simply changing what time of the day you take your other medicines in conjunction with the doctor recommended thyroid medicine. It is also possible that certain foods could end up being involved in the efficacy of your thyroid medicine. It is best to discuss all of this with your doctor to come up with an efficient way for you to take your thyroid medicine, based on your dietary needs.

The severity of complications due to leaving Hashimoto's untreated varies and are not worth the risk if you ever contract, or if you have it. They go far beyond just hypothyroidism and include heart problems that an include total failure of the heart. It is not unusual for anemia to be a result of leaving Hashimoto's disease unattended. Depression and a decrease in libido are common, as well as higher levels of cholesterol in the blood and experiencing a sense of confusion or loss of consciousness.

Hashimoto's disease has also been the culprit responsible for complications during a woman's pregnancy cycle. It is far more likely, that if you carry out a pregnancy while having untreated Hashimoto's disease, that you may be putting your child at higher risk of being born with defects of their kidneys, their heart, and even their brains.

These complications can be limited by talking to your doctor during the pregnancy and keeping on top of monitoring your thyroid glands hormone levels with the proper blood testing. If you are a pregnant woman and have thyroid issues, such preventative measures could mean a severe change in the life and health of your child. However, if you have not had any known disorders with your thyroid or hormone levels, it is not recommended that you get regular or constant screening done during the pregnancy.

Graves' Disease

Another autoimmune disorder, Graves' disease is responsible for causing your thyroid gland too create too much of the thyroid hormones in your body. When this happens it is a condition referred to commonly as hyperthyroidism. Graves' disease, is named such for the man who discovered it, an Irish physician named Robert J. Graves, and is regarded as one of the most common forms hyperthyroidism takes, having an effect on around 1 out of every 200 people.

When Graves' disease occurs in the body, it will cause your immune system to begin creating antibodies that are known as thyroid-stimulating immunoglobulins, that attach themselves to the body's usually healthy cells of the thyroid gland. By doing this they end up causing the thyroid gland to produce and secrete more of the thyroid hormones than it is meant to for your body. The hormones that are produced by the thyroid gland go on to affect a great number of your body's functions including its temperature, the function of the nervous system, the development of the brain, and the list goes on. For this reason, hyperthyroidism can end up having a negatively driven affect on not just all of those functions, but when left untreated can also cause the loss of weight and mental and physical fatigue. Hyperthyroidism has also been found to be responsible for such things as depression and emotional liability where the individual will uncontrollably cry or laugh or put on other manic emotional displays.

Due to the role that Graves' disease can invariably play on the appearance of hyperthyroidism in the body, it is no surprise that the two would contain a sharing of many of the same symptoms. These symptoms include tremors especially of the hands, a loss of weight, tachycardia, which is the rapidity in the rate of the heart, becoming intolerant to heat or warmth, fatigue, nervousness and irritability, the swelling of the front of the neck, due to the enlargement of the thyroid gland, known as a goiter, an increase in the frequency of having bowel movements, as well as diarrhea, weakness of the muscles, and having it become difficult to get a good full night's worth of sleep. Among the people who experience having Graves' disease, it is only a small percentage who will experience the skin thickening around their shin area and become reddened, an affliction which is known as Graves' dermopathy.

Another common symptom of Graves' disease which one may go through while experiencing the condition, is what is called Graves' ophthalmopathy. Graves' ophthalmopathy is what occurs when the eyes of the afflicted individual appear to be enlarged, which is a result of the eyelids retracting. When Graves' ophthalmopathy happens, it is entirely possible that your eyes may begin to bulge outwards from your eye sockets.

Estimates say that as much as 30 percent of the people who end up developing Graves' disease will observe at least a mild case of what is known as Graves' ophthalmopathy and that for up to 5 percent of the people will instead experience an extreme case of the eye bulging.

Because of autoimmune diseases such as Graves' disease, the immune system will begin to fight against what are the healthy cells and healthy tissues of the body. Normally, your immune system is producing proteins which are known as antibodies, which are responsible for fighting against foreign invaders to your body, the likes of harmful viruses and bacteria. The antibodies produced this way are formed especially with the duty of targeting a specific invader to the host. When it comes to the effect of Graves' disease on the body, your immune system begins to mistake healthy thyroid cells as these foreign harmful cells and produces the thyroid-stimulating immunoglobulins which then mistakenly go off to attack what are your healthy thyroid cells.

Scientists and doctors alike, are aware that it is indeed possible for a person to have inherited the ability for their body to make antibodies which then go against their own healthy cells, yet they have made no determination that such an occurrence is what is the cause for Graves' disease, or who will end up developing Graves' disease.

Despite that though, there are experts who believe that they have been able to button down on some factors which may increase ones risk for the development of graves disease which includes its tendency to be hereditary. So be sure to discuss family medical history with your doctor and talk about whether or not there are family members who have, or who ay have had Graves' disease. It is also believed by these experts that stress, gender, and someone's age may be some of the facets that end up putting someone at higher risk of getting Graves' disease. It is typical for the disease to be found in people who are younger than the age of 40, and it has been more prevalent, about seven to eight times so, in women rather than men.

Having had, or having still, another autoimmune disease is yet another factor that will increase your risk of ever getting Graves' disease. Examples of such autoimmune diseases are having Crohn's disease, rheumatoid arthritis, and diabetes mellitus, among others.

For the diagnosing of Graves' disease, when it is suspected, it is not unheard of for your doctor to request lab tests. The use of your families medical history as well, especially if there is a case of someone in your family having had Graves' disease, will be able to help act as a basis for your doctor to zero in on diagnosing whether you have Graves' disease as well or not. This is something that thyroid gland blood tests will be needed for in order to confirm. Your doctor may request that these tests and others may be handled by a specialist expert in diseases which are related to the body's hormones, known as an endocrinologist, in order to help get the diagnosis of Graves' disease. Other tests which your doctor may request are full bloodwork tests, a thyroid gland scan, an uptake test utilizing radioactive iodine, a test for levels of TSH, or thyroid stimulating hormone, and a TSI test, which is the thyroid-stimulating immunoglobulins.

By combining the efforts of the endocrinologist, as well as the array of tests, it is more possible for your doctor to determine if you do indeed have and need treatment for Graves' disease specifically, or if another thyroid disorder is what is at work, and thus requires its own specific form of treatment.

There are a number of options available for treatment when someone is diagnosed as having Graves' disease. These are generally the taking of anti-thyroid drugs, therapy in the form of RAI, or radioactive iodine, and getting thyroid gland surgery. It is not abnormal for a doctor, in the case of Graves' disease, to recommend, all, two, or just one of the treatments for the afflicted.

When it comes to treatment via anti-thyroid drugs, you will typically be taking medications such as methimazole, which is taken orally as a tablet and works by putting a stop to the thyroid gland producing and secreting too much thyroid hormone, and propylthiouracil, which is also taken orally and generally used as a back up if a drug like methimazole did not end up working well enough. The use of beta-blockers is also recommended on occasion as they are used in assistance of reducing the effects of symptoms until another treatment method can start working.

It is radioactive iodine treatment, or RAI, which is among the most common treatments suggested to those suffering of Graves' disease. It is required, during this treatment, that the individual seeking treatment take specified doses of radioactive iodine-131, the purpose of which is to destroy thyroid cells. The radioactive iodine-131 will be ingested orally, in small amounts, via pill. Be sure to discuss with your doctor and risks or precautions that come with this treatment.

The less frequent option for treatment is the thyroid surgery. This treatment will tend to be a last resort if the other options have not worked to full capacity, if there is a reason to be suspect of thyroid cancer being present, or if the patient is a pregnant woman who is unable to take any of the regularly prescribed anti-thyroid drugs.

In the case of surgery being necessary, it is not uncommon the doctor to issue the removal of your thyroid gland completely, in the interest of preventing the return of the hyperthyroidism. In which case, thyroid hormone replacement surgery will be necessary on a regular basis. Talk to your doctor about the possible side effects of choosing to go through with surgery, as well as generally what to expect moving forward.

Goiter

A goiter, goitre, thyroid cyst, or Plummer's disease, is a general term used for when there is an observable enlargement of the thyroid gland, usually resulting in a noticeable swelling of the front of the neck. Treatment for a goiter can be handled in a variety of ways, and the treatment method is dependent on the goiters location, the length of its presence, and how exactly it is affecting the thyroid glands performance.

Though usually unable to be seen or even felt, the thyroid gland generally tends to become detectable by touch and even perceptible to the eye when there is a goiter present. An expanse of the thyroid gland, or goiter, can be the cause of the whole thyroid gland expanding, which is known as a "smooth goiter", or just a part of the thyroid gland expanding, which is also called a "cystic" or "nodular" goiter. A goiter is not a sure symptom of having an active thyroid, known as hyperthyroidism, or underactive thyroid, known as hypothyroidism, and, in fact, the majority of people who have a goiter, retain a perfectly normal use of their thyroid gland.

A number of reasons exist for the existence of a goiter. Among these are included a deficiency in your levels of iodine. Iodine may be a trace element, but it is far from trivial. It assists in helping the thyroid gland in maintaining proper functionality and making the thyroid glands hormones. There are two primary hormones which are produced and secreted by the thyroid gland, these are T4 or thyroxine, and T3, also known as triiodothyronine. The approximate number of people who have iodine deficiency comes out to about 2.2 billion and it is estimated that around 29 percent of the worlds total population live in an area that is considered to be deficient in iodine. It is reported that people in the U.K. have proper levels of iodine as a part of their regular diet. If you are keeping your eye out for food sources that are a good source of iodine, there are salts that have iodine supplements, as well, non-organic milk is plentiful with iodine.

Thyroiditis is anther well known cause of goiter. Thyroiditis is more commonly referred to as when the thyroid gland has become inflamed. Around the world, the most common reason for thyroiditis occurring is Hashimoto's disease, or Hashimoto's thyroiditis, which is an autoimmune disease that causes the bodies antibodies to start to become confused and begin attacking healthy cells of the thyroid gland. Hashimoto's disease is not the only cause of the thyroiditis condition though, it could also stem from viral infection, and has been known to occur just after or during pregnancy.

A goiter has also been known to occur due to Graves' disease, another autoimmune disease, this one causing the immune systems antibodies attacks on thyroid cells to make the thyroid gland overactive, resulting in hyperthyroidism. It is this hyperthyroidism, or over activity of the thyroid glands capacity for producing and secreting hormones, which is the cause of the swelling of the thyroid gland.

If there are benign growths on the thyroid gland, they have been known to cause a goiter, most commonly known for doing this is a follicular adenoma, which can be a firm or rubbery tumor surrounded by a fibrous capsule.

External factors that may be the cause of goiter are known as goitrogens. Included among what would be considered a goitrogen are medicines such as the mental health drug lithium, and cabbage type vegetables. Ingestion in the excess of these vegetables, which include cassava or kelp, will likely result in the growth formation of a goiter.

There are physiological demands put on the body during pregnancy and during puberty which have been known to be at the root of a goiter. And as with other causes like Graves' disease and Hashimoto's disease, there is a strong likelihood of inherited genetic reasons that one may at some point experience goiter.

Due to the varying reasons for the existence of goiter, there are also a multiplicity of types of goiter. The first of these types is known as colloid goiter, or endemic goiter, which is a development due directly to a lack of sufficient iodine levels. As a result, the people who tend to end up with a colloid goiter are those we mentioned, who live somewhere with a less dense supply of iodine.

The next type of goiter is the nontoxic goiter, or sporadic goiter, as it is also well known. Though the definite cause of a goiter of this type is regarded as generally unknown, it is surmised that a sporadic goiter is a result of taking medications, such as lithium, for example, or so it is believed. Among the may uses for lithium, it is perhaps most commonly recognized as the drug used for aiding in the treatment of mood based disorders, the likes of bipolar or depression. The nontoxic name is apt in regard to this form of goiter, as they are benign, and have no discernable effect on the production or secretion function of the thyroid gland, leaving the thyroid to function at a healthy and normal capacity.

The final type of commonly recognized goiter is known as the toxic nodular or multinodular goiter. Generally originating and taking form from as merely an extension from what was a simple goiter prior, the toxic nodular goiter will take the form of at least one, but often more, small nodules on the expanding thyroid gland. This toxic nodular goiter, having taken a sort of root on the thyroid gland, then begins to produce its own thyroid hormone, which plays a big part in the causation of hyperthyroidism.

As mentioned above, it can be difficult to detect goiter before it has really taken effect to the thyroid gland, but after it has begun doing it's work it is most common for it to cause a swelling of the front of the neck, making it clearly visible as well as felt. Before the expanding has commenced, it is common to have had nodules existing in your thyroid gland, these small nodules cannot be felt, and may have even been only a chance occurrence due to examinations, and of scans, that were applied for other reasons. Cases such as these are rather common, and when they occur, there has been a tendency to notice no sign of a goiter up to that point. As nodules appear on the thyroid, ranging from smaller nodules to much larger nodules, it is the presence of these nodules which is what is the cause of noticeable swelling of the neck.

This swelling and the nodules which are collecting on the thyroid gland cause other symptoms to occur, like having a difficult time of swallowing or of trying to breathe, it is not uncommon for coughing to be a symptom, your voice may start to become hoarse, and there may be a dizzy sensation that is noticeable when you raise an arm above your head.

Goiter is a rather common occurrence. It is calculated by the World Health Organization, that around the world, goiter affects nearly 12 percent of the global population. However, it has also been recorded that in Europe, the rate of goiter is lower by a slight amount. Goiter being considered endemic, or noticeably affecting a certain area is a common occurrence wherever iodine is scarce, and the endemic definitions are only applied when goiter is recognized on 1 out of 10 people within a certain population.

It is usual for goiter to be the diagnosis when there is noticeable swelling on the neck that can be seen without the need of a scan, also making it detectable with the touch of the hand, due to the enlarged thyroid gland in your neck, something a doctor will be quick to check for, likely before anything else.

There are also a number tests a general practitioner may order in order to examine the levels in your blood of thyroid hormones coming from the thyroid gland, as well as wanting to make sure of the levels of antibodies that are prevalent in the bloodstream. This examination will often take the form of blood tests, that are used to detect the changes in levels of the hormones as well as whether or not the level of production of the antibodies has increased, which tends to happen in response to the body experiencing an injury or infection in the blood.

A thyroid scan, or thyroid uptake scan, will show the size of the goiter itself, as well as what condition the goiter is in. It will also aid in identifying any differences in activity, in various places on the thyroid gland.

A biopsy may be recommended, the procedure of which involves removing samples of your thyroid gland, and then sending the samples of your thyroid gland's tissue to an outside laboratory or endocrinologist for examination.

It is also possible that an ultrasound scan may be used which will help for a doctor to see images of the inside of your neck, getting a much closer look at the size of the invasive goiter, allowing for the observation of nodules. As more ultrasounds are done, it is even then possible to track the changes in size or shape of the nodules, and the size of the goiter.

You may, at some point, be referred to an endocrinologist in order to get an outpatient assessment, giving you and the doctor more information from the examination by an expert. During their examination you may have to undergo a test known as a fine needle aspiration, which is done on the thyroid gland. For the procedure to take place, the endocrinologist will make use of a fine needle which, utilizing the guiding sight of an ultrasound, will be used to remove tissue from your thyroid gland, only a small amount will be needed. The tissue removed from your thyroid gland is then studied under the lens of a microscope, which will assist the endocrinologist in assessing exactly the types of cells which are currently present in your thyroid gland. It is not at all uncommon for a procedure like this to need to be repeated one or more times, for the sake of reaching an accurate result and helping you on your way to treatment and recovery.

There is no one, cut and dry, blanket method for treating a goiter, as the treatment will depend entirely on precisely what is the cause that is underlying the goiter. As well, a particular course of action will be decided by your doctor on the basis of the size of the goiter, and the condition that the goiter is in, as well as the symptoms you have that are associated with the goiter. It will also be important to not overlook any factors to your health that may have been responsible for the goiters formation when looking into treatment options.

A goiter which can be regarded as simple, having a prevalence of causing no imbalances in the thyroid gland, as well as no seeming problems as a result of the thyroid gland, will be less likely to cause further obstructions or overall issues.

In order to shrink a goiter, in the case of hypo or hyperthyroidism, it may be enough to just take prescribed medicines as a treatment for the symptoms and for the swelling of the thyroid gland. Medications which are known as corticosteroids often see use in the task of reducing any inflammation, or when there is a prevalence of thyroiditis.

Medicinal treatments for a goiter are not always the most effective response, however. It is not at all uncommon for a goiter to have grown too large to be able to respond properly to medicinal therapy and begin to shrink. In such a case there are surgeries which are available, known as a thyroidectomy. Undergoing a thyroidectomy will mean removing your thyroid gland completely and is a common option for when the thyroid gland grows too large and further obstructs what would otherwise be simple actions, such as swallowing or breathing.

When you are going through the experience of trying to treat what is the most harmful of the goiter family, the toxic nodular or multinodular goiter, RAI, or radioactive iodine treatment is typically the necessary response. You will be given a tablet, the RAI, which is a small amount of the radioactive iodine, which gets ingested orally and begins the process of destroying thyroid gland tissue.

When it comes to the treatment of a goiter, there are options for home care which can be very helpful and ought not to be overlooked as such. When you have finished up with all the treatment that can be offered at the hospital, or by a referred endocrinologist, it is an entirely common possibility that a discussion with your general practitioner will end in him or her suggesting you continue care of yourself in the home, with a prescription of some form of medication, which may end up being a decrease or increase in the amounts of iodine that you are ingesting regularly. This will, of course, be determined by the type of goiter that was ailing you, as well as requiring regular testing to keep an eye on your iodine levels, and the efficiency of your thyroid glands production and secretion of hormones. If it all ends up that a goiter is non-problematic, being too small to count as an issue or cause an imbalance, you may require no treatment or care at home at all.

PART III

Hormone Diet

Are you worried that your hormones are not at their optimal levels? Here is a diet that will solve your problems.

Chapter 1: Health Benefits of the Hormone Diet

When it comes to getting healthy through weight loss, there's never any shortage of fitness crazes and diets that claim to have the secret to easy and sustainable weight loss. One of the latest diet plans that have come into the spotlight is the hormone diet, which claims that people often struggle to lose weight because of their hormones.

A hormone diet is a 3-step process that spans over six weeks and is designed to synchronize your hormones and promote a healthy body through detoxification, nutritional supplements, exercise, and diet. The diet controls what you eat and informs you about the correct time to eat to ensure maximum benefits to your hormones. Many books have been written on this topic with supporters of the diet assuring people that they can lose weight quickly and significantly through diet and exercise and reset or manipulate their hormones. Although the diet has a few variations, the central idea around each is that correcting the body's perceived hormonal imbalances is the key to losing weight.

The most important benefit of a hormone diet is that it takes a solid stance on improving overall health through weight loss and promoting regular exercise as well as natural, nutritious foods. Apart from that, it also focuses on adequate sleep, stress management, emotional health, and other healthy lifestyle habits that are all essential components that people should follow, whether it's a part of a diet or not. Including a water diet, it aims towards losing about twelve pounds in the 1st phase and 2 pounds a week after that.

Hormones have an essential role in the body's everyday processes, like helping bones grow, digesting food, etc. They act as "chemical messengers," instructing the cells to perform specific actions and are transported around the body through the bloodstream.

One of the very important food items to be included in the hormone diet is salmon. Salmon is rich in omega-3 fatty acids, Docosahexaenoic acid, and Eicosapentaenoic acid (EPA). It is rich in selenium too. These help to lower your blood pressure and also reduce the level of unhealthy cholesterol in the blood. These make you less prone to heart diseases. Salmon is a rich source of healthy fat. If consumed in sufficient amounts, it provides you energy and helps you get rid of unwanted body fat. Salmon is well-known for giving fantastic weight loss results as it has less saturated fat, unlike other protein sources. Salmon is packed with vitamins like vitamin-k, E, D, and A. These are extremely helpful for your eyes, bone joints, etc. These vitamins are also good for your brain, regulation of metabolic balance, and repairing your muscles. Salmon's vitamins and omega-3 fatty acids are amazing for sharpening your mind. It also improves your memory retention power. If you consume salmon, you are less likely to develop dementia or mental dis-functions. Salmon has anti-inflammatory properties and is low in omega-6 fatty acid content (which is pro-inflammatory in nature and is present in a huge amount in the modern diet). It promotes healthy skin and gives you radiant and glowing skin. It is good for the winter because it helps you to stay warm. It also provides lubrication to your joints because of the abundant presence of essential minerals and fatty acids in it. Apart from this, some other things to include in your diet are arugula, kale, ginger, avocado, carrots, and so on.

There are almost sixteen hormones that can influence weight. For example, the hormone leptin produced by your fat cells is considered a "satiety hormone," which makes you feel full by reducing your appetite. As a signaling hormone, it communicates with the part of your brain (hypothalamus) that controls food intake and appetite. Leptin informs the brain when there is enough fat in storage, and extra fat is not required. This helps prevent overeating. Individuals who are obese or overweight generally have very high levels of leptin in their blood. Research shows that the level of leptin in obese individuals was almost four times higher than that in individuals with normal weight.

Studies have found that fat hormones like leptin and adiponectin can promote long-term weight loss by reducing appetite and increasing metabolism. It is believed that both these fat hormones follow the same pathway in the brain to manage blood sugar (glucose) and body weight (Robert V. Considine, 1996).

Simply put, the hormone diet works by helping to create a calorie deficit through better nutritional habits and exercise, which ultimately results in weight loss. It's also essential to consult a doctor before following this detox diet or consuming any dietary supplements.

Chapter 2: Hormone-Rebalancing Smoothies

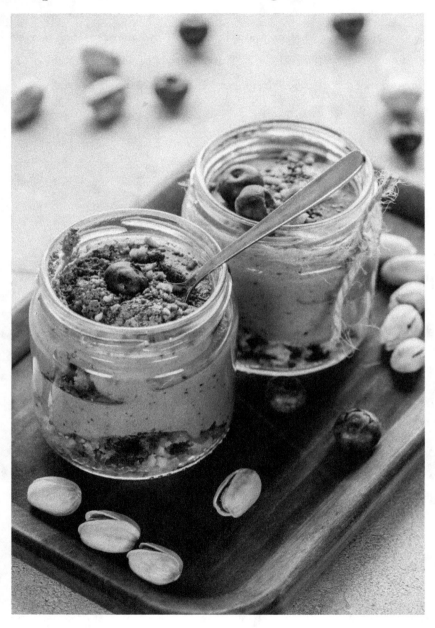

Estrogen Detox Smoothie

Total Prep & Cooking Time: 5 minutes

Yields: One glass

Nutrition Facts: Calories: 312 | Carbs: 47.9g | Protein: 18.6g | Fat: 8.5g | Fiber: 3g

Ingredients:

- Half a cup of hemp seeds
- Two kiwis (medium-sized)
- A quarter each of
  - Avocado (medium-sized)
  - Cucumber (medium-sized)
- Half a unit each of
  - Lemon (squeezed freshly)
  - Green apple
- One celery (medium-sized)
- A quarter cup of cilantro
- Two tbsps. of chis seeds
- Two cups of water (filtered)
- One tsp. of cacao nibs
- One tbsp. of coconut oil

Method:

1. Blend the ingredients all together to form a smoothie at high speed. The thickness can be adjusted according to your preference by adding more water to the mixture.

2. Serve and enjoy.

Dopamine Delight Smoothie

Total Prep Time: 10 minutes

Yields: One serving

Nutrition Facts: Calories: 383 | Carbs: 31g | Protein: 24g | Fat: 18.g | Fiber: 3g

Ingredients:

- Half a teaspoon of cinnamon (ground)
- Half a cup of peeled banana (the bananas must be frozen)
- One organic espresso, double shot (measuring half a cup)
- One tablespoon of chia seeds
- A three-fourth cup of soy milk (plain or vanilla-flavored)
- Protein powder, a serving (from the whey with the flavor of vanilla)

Method:

1. Fill in the bowl of your blender with all the ingredients (from the section of ingredients) except the whey protein powder and then proceed by switching to a high-speed blending option. Make sure it acquires a smooth consistency and then pour it out.

2. Now you may add the protein powder and give it another shot of blend until the whole things get incorporated, a bit of the goat cheese (already crumbled).

Breakfast Smoothie Bowl

Total Prep Time: 10 minutes

Yields: 2 servings

Nutrition Facts: Calories: 290 | Carbs: 53g | Protein: 6g | Fat: 8g | Fiber: 9g

Ingredients:

- One cup of thoroughly rinsed blueberries (fresh and ripe)
- A sundry of nuts and fruits for garnishing, which includes – strawberries, bananas (thinly sliced), peanuts (Spanish), kiwi (chopped), segments of tangerine, and raspberries.
- One cup of Greek yogurt

For the preparation of honey flax granola,

- Two tablespoons each of
  - Flaxseeds
  - Vegetable oil
- Oats (old-fashioned), approximately a cup
- One tablespoon of honey

Method:

1. Set your oven at a temperature of 350 degrees F.

2. Preparation of the smoothie: collect the diverse types of berries, wash them thoroughly, and then put them in the blender and turn it on. Make an even mixture out of it. Add some amount of the yogurt and blend it again to form a smooth texture.

3. For preparing the granola: Take a small-sized bowl and then drizzle a few drops oil in it. Then add the oats, flax, and honey to the oil, one by one, and mix it well. You are required to toss the bowl thoroughly to get the mixture well-coated with the poured oil. After you are done, place the oats mixture in a baking sheet evenly. Bake it for about twenty minutes. This mark will be enough to give the oats a beautiful tinge of golden brown. Allow it to cool.

4. Now you will require a shallow bowl to spoon in some yogurt, and this will be the first layer. Form a second layer with the various fruits and nuts and finally for the third layer, top with the granola.

5. Enjoy.

Notes:

- *Using frozen nuts and fruits in a warm-weather will get much to your relief.*

- *For a vegan smoothie bowl, sub the yogurt with coconut or almond yogurt.*

- *Give the pan a few strokes while baking the oats.*

Blueberry Detox Smoothie

Total Prep Time: Ten minutes

Yields: One serving

Nutrition Facts: Calories: 326 | Carbs: 65g | Protein: 4g | Fat: 8g | Fiber: 9g

Ingredients:

- One cup of wild blueberries (frozen)
- One banana (sliced into several pieces) frozen
- Orange juice (approximately half a cup)
- Cilantro leaves, fresh (approximately a measuring a small handful size)
- A quarter of an entire avocado
- A quarter cup of water

Method:

1. Add cilantro, avocado, water, blueberries, banana, and orange juice in the blender and then process.

2. Make the ingredients integrated so well that they become smooth in their consistency.

Notes: *It is recommended that you add the potent herb, cilantro, or parsley in a small amount when consuming this smoothie for the first time, as it might trigger a mild headache. If you do not get a headache, you may add a bit more of the cilantro leaves.*

Maca Mango Smoothie

Total Prep & Cooking Time: 2 minutes

Yields: 2 servings

Nutrition Facts: Calories: 53 | Carbs: 13g | Protein: 1g | Fat: 3g | Fiber: 1.5g

Ingredients:

- One and a half cups each of
  - Fresh mango
  - Frozen mango
- One tablespoon each of
  - Ground flaxseed
  - Nut butter
- One teaspoon of ground turmeric
- Two teaspoons of maca root powder
- Three-quarter cups of nut milk
- One frozen banana

Method:

1. Blend all the ingredients together to get a smooth mixture.

2. Adjust consistency by adding nut milk.

3. Once done, divide into two glasses and enjoy!

Pituitary Relief Smoothie

Total Prep & Cooking Time: 5 minutes

Yields: 2 servings

Nutrition Facts: Calories: 174 | Carbs: 18.3g | Protein: 9.7g | Fat: 8.3g | Fiber: 14.4g

Ingredients:

- One teaspoon of coconut oil
- One fresh or frozen ripe banana
- One tablespoon of raw sesame seeds
- Two teaspoons each of
  o Chia seeds
  o Raw Maca powder
  o Raw Spirulina
- Two cups of water
- Two tablespoons of hulled hemp seeds

Method:

1. You have to use a blender to process this smoothie. Add the hulled hemp seeds, sesame seeds, and water in the blender and process them. Do it at high speed, and it will only require a minute. This will give you raw-milk like texture.

2. Then, add the following ingredients into it – coconut oil, banana, chia seeds, Maca, and Spirulina, and process the ingredients once again but this time on medium speed for another minute or so. Everything will become well incorporated.

3. You have to drink this smoothie on an empty stomach.

Notes: *In order to make the smoothie rich in antioxidants, you can add some fresh fruits like blueberries, kiwi, and raspberries.*

Chapter 2: Easy Breakfast Recipes

Scrambled Eggs With Feta and Tomatoes

Total Prep & Cooking Time: 10 minutes

Yields: One Plate

Nutrition Facts: Calories: 421 | Carbs: 8.6g | Protein: 20.3g | Fat: 35.1g | Fiber: 1.6g

Ingredients:

- One tbsp. each of
  - Olive oil (extra virgin)
  - Freshly chopped parsley, basil, dill or chives
- Half a cup of cherry tomatoes (each tomato sliced into half)
- Two ounces of crumbled feta cheese (approximately a quarter cup)
- Two eggs are beaten
- Two tbsp. of onion (diced)
- To taste:
  - Black pepper
  - Kosher salt

Method:

1. Keep the beaten eggs in a small-sized bowl and then season it with a pinch of pepper and salt. Set the bowl aside.

2. Use a nonstick skillet to proceed with the cooking. Pour two tbsp. of olive oil. Then add the diced onions. Stir over moderate heat and cook until softened. Make sure that the onions do not look brown. This process should get done by a minute.

3. Add half a cup of tomatoes to skillet and then continue to mix for about two minutes.

4. Now you may add the eggs. Using a spatula, gather the beaten eggs to the center by moving spatula all over the skillet.

5. The eggs will take an additional minute to get cooked. So after that mark, add the parsley or other herbs (if preferred) and feta cheese. Keep the eggs underdone as they will get cooked completely after they are served in the plate itself (from the residual heat). Therefore, cook the entire thing in the skillet for 30 seconds only.

6. Take a serving plate and transfer the eggs to it. Top with some sprinkled parsley and feta cheese, drizzled with some oil, and seasoned with some pepper and salt. These additions are optional and may vary as per your desire.

Smashed Avo and Quinoa

Total Prep & Cooking Time: 15 minutes

Yields: Six bowls

Nutrition Facts: Calories: 492 | Carbs: 67g | Protein: 15g | Fat: 20g | Fiber: 13g

Ingredients:

- One avocado skinned, cut into half, and then pitted
- A handful of cilantro or coriander
- Half a lemon (juiced)
- A quarter red onion (diced finely)
- One-eighth teaspoon of cayenne pepper
- To taste: Sea salt

For the Greens,

- One handful of kale
- One handful of soft herbs (basil, parsley or mint)
- One handful of chard or spinach
- For frying: butter or coconut oil

Serve with,

- One cup of quinoa (cooked)

Method:

1. You will require a frying pan to get this done. To it, add the coconut oil or butter (whichever you prefer) and add the greens. Toss them carefully and then sauté over moderate heat. Stop when they become soft.

2. Mix the onion, cayenne, avocado, cilantro, salt, lemon, and pepper to a bowl and mix them completely. The pepper and salt must be added according to the taste.

3. Add cooked quinoa to the tossed greens and heat altogether over low heat.

4. Take a serving plate and place the quinoa mixture and greens to it. Crown the whole thing with smashed avocado and then serve.

Hormone Balancing Granola

Total Prep & Cooking Time: 35 minutes

Yields: 8 servings

Nutrition Facts: Calories: 360 | Carbs: 19.8g | Protein: 5.1g | Fat: 28.8g | Fiber: 5.8g

Ingredients:

- One-third cup each of
  - Flaxseed meal
  - Pumpkin seeds
  - Seedless raisins
- Two teaspoons of cinnamon
- One teaspoon of vanilla extract
- Four tablespoons of maple syrup
- Five tablespoons of melted coconut oil
- A quarter cup of unsweetened coconut flakes
- Two-thirds cup each of
  - Chopped pecans
  - Chopped brazil nuts
- Two tablespoons of ground chia seeds

Method:

1. Set the temperature of the oven to 180 degrees F and preheat.

2. In a food processor, chop the pecans and the Brazil nuts. Then, mix these chopped nuts with coconut flakes, seeds, and other nuts present in the list of ingredients.

3. Add maple syrup, coconut oil, cinnamon, and vanilla extract in a separate bowl and combine well.

4. Now, take the wet ingredients and pour them into the dry ingredients. Mix thoroughly so that everything has become coated properly.

5. Place the prepared mixture in the oven for half an hour and cook.

6. Once done, cut into pieces and serve.

Chapter 3: Healthy Lunch Recipes

Easy Shakshuka

Total Prep & Cooking Time: 30 minutes

Yields: Six servings

Nutrition Facts: Calories: 154 | Carbs: 4.1g | Protein: 9g | Fat: 7.8g | Fiber: 0g

Ingredients:

- Olive oil (extra virgin)
- Two chopped green peppers
- One teaspoon each of
  - Paprika (sweet)
  - Coriander (ground)
- A pinch of red pepper (flakes)
- Half a cup of tomato sauce
- A quarter cup each of
  - Mint leaves (freshly chopped)
  - Parsley leaves (chopped freshly)
- One yellow onion, large-sized (chopped)
- Two cloves of garlic, chopped
- Half a teaspoon of cumin (ground)
- Six cups of chopped tomatoes (Vine-ripe)
- Six large-sized eggs

- To taste: Pepper and salt

Method:

1. You will require a large-sized skillet (made of cast iron). Pour three tablespoons of oil and heat it. After bringing the oil to boil, add the peppers, spices, onions, garlic, pepper, and salt. Stir time to time to cook the veggies for five minutes until they become softened.

2. After the vegetables become soft, add the chopped tomatoes and then tomato sauce. Cover the skillet and simmer for an additional fifteen minutes.

3. Now, you may remove the lid from the pan and then cook a touch more to thicken the consistency. At this point, you may adjust the taste.

4. Make six cavities within the tomato mixture and crack one egg each inside the cavities.

5. Cover the skillet after reducing the heat and allow it to cook so that the eggs settle into the cavities.

6. Keep track of the time and accordingly uncover the skillet and then add mint and parsley. Season with more black and red pepper according to your desire. Serve them warm with the sort of bread you wish.

Ginger Chicken

Total Prep & Cooking Time: 50 minutes

Yields: Six Servings

Nutrition Facts: Calories: 310 | Carbs: 6g | Protein: 37g | Fat: 16g | Fiber: 1g

Ingredients:

- A one-kilogram pack of chicken thighs (skinless and boneless)
- Four cloves of garlic (chopped finely)
- A fifteen-gram pack of coriander (fresh and chopped)
- Two tablespoons of sunflower oil
- One teaspoon each of
  - Turmeric (ground)
  - Chili powder (mild)
- A four hundred milliliter can of coconut milk (reduced-fat)
- One cube of chicken stock
- One ginger properly peeled and chopped finely (it should be of the size of a thumb)
- One lime, juiced
- Two medium-sized onions
- One red chili, sliced and the seeds removed (fresh)

Method:

1. Make the chicken thighs into three large chunks and marinate them with chili powder, garlic, coriander (half of the entire amount), ginger, oil (one tbsp.), and lime juice. Cover the bowl after stirring them well and then store it in the fridge until oven-ready.

2. Marinade the chicken and keep overnight for better flavor.

3. Chop the onions finely (it is going to be the simplest for preparing the curry) before dropping them into the food processor. Pour oil into the frying pan (large-sized) and heat it. Then add chopped onions and stir them thoroughly for eight minutes until the pieces become soft. Then pour the turmeric powder and stir for an additional minute.

4. Now add the chicken mixture and cook on high heat until you notice a change in its color. Pour the chicken stock, chili, and coconut milk and after covering the pan simmer for another twenty minutes. Sprinkle the left-over coriander leaves and then serve hot.

5. Enjoy.

Carrot and Miso Soup

Total Prep & Cooking Time: 1 hour

Yields: Four bowls of soup

Nutrition Facts: Calories: 76 | Carbs: 8.76g | Protein: 4.83g | Fat: 2.44g | Fiber: 1.5g

Ingredients:

- Two tbsps. of oil
- Garlic, minced (four cloves)
- One inch of garlic (grated)
- Three tbsps. of miso paste (white)
- One diced onion
- One pound of carrot (sliced thinly)
- Four cups of vegetable stock
- To taste: Pepper and Salt

For garnishing,

- Two scallions (sliced thinly)
- Chili pepper (seven spices)
- One nori roasted (make thin slivers)
- Sesame oil

Method:

1. Using a soup pot will be convenient to proceed with. Pour oil in a pot and then heat over a high flame. Now you may put garlic, carrot, and onion and sauté them thoroughly. Cook for about ten minutes so that the onions turn translucent.

2. Then add the ginger and vegetable stock. Mix them well and cook all together. Put the flame to simmer. Cover the pot while cooking to make the carrot tender. This will take another thirty minutes.

3. Put off the flame and puree the soup with the help of an immersion blender.

4. Use a small-sized bowl to whisk together a spoonful of the soup and the white miso paste. Stir until the paste dissolve and pour the mixture back to the pot.

5. Add pepper and salt if required.

6. Divide the soup among four bowls and enrich its feel by adding scallions, sesame oil, seven spices, and nori.

Arugula Salad

Total Prep & Cooking Time: 1 hour 10 minutes

Yields: Two bowls of salad

Nutrition Facts: Calories: 336.8 | Carbs: 30.6g | Protein: 7.7g | Fat: 22.2g | Fiber: 7.3g

Ingredients:

For the salad,

- Two medium-sized beets (boiled or roasted for about an hour), skinned and sliced into pieces that can easily be bitten
- Four tablespoons of goat cheese
- Approximately 2.5 oz. of baby arugula (fresh)
- A quarter cup of walnuts (chopped roughly before toasting)

For the dressing,

- Three tablespoons of olive oil (extra virgin)
- A quarter tsp. each of
   o Mustard powder (dried)
   o Pepper
- Half a tsp. each of
   o Salt
   o Sugar

- One and a half tablespoons of lemon juice

Method:

1. For preparing the vinaigrette, place all the ingredients (listed in the dressing ingredients section) in a jar and then shake them to emulsify. At this stage, before starting with the process of emulsification, you may add or remove the ingredients as per your liking.

2. Get the salad assembled (again depending upon the taste you want to give it), add a fistful of arugula leaves, place some chopped beets (after they have been cooked), and finally the toasted walnuts (already chopped).

3. Drizzle vinaigrette over the salad and enjoy.

Notes:

- *Coat the beets with oil (olive), roll them up in an aluminum foil, and then roast the beets at a temperature of 400 degrees F.*

- *And for boiling the beets, immerse them in water after transferring to a pot and simmer them for 45 minutes.*

Kale Soup

Total Prep & Cooking Time: 55 minutes

Yields: 8 servings

Nutrition Facts: Calories: 277.3 | Carbs: 50.9g | Protein: 9.6g | Fat: 4.5g | Fiber: 10.3g

Ingredients:

- Two tbsps. of dried parsley
- One tbsp. of Italian seasoning
- Salt and pepper
- Thirty oz. of drained cannellini beans
- Six peeled and cubed white potatoes
- Fifteen ounces of diced tomatoes
- Six vegetable Bouillon cubes
- Eight cups of water
- One bunch of kale (with chopped leaves and stems removed)
- Two tbsps. of chopped garlic
- One chopped yellow onion
- Two tbsps. of olive oil

Method:

1. At first, take a large soup pot, add in some olive oil, and heat it.

2. Add garlic and onion. Cook them until soft.

3. Then stir in the kale and cook for about two minutes, until wilted.

4. Pour the water and add the beans, potatoes, tomatoes, vegetable bouillon, parsley, and the Italian seasoning.

5. On medium heat, simmer the soup for about twenty-five minutes, until the potatoes are cooked through.

6. Finally, do the seasoning with salt and pepper according to your taste.

Roasted Sardines

Total Prep & Cooking Time: 25 minutes

Yields: 4 servings

Nutrition Facts: Calories: 418 | Carbs: 2.6g | Protein: 41g | Fat: 27.2g | Fiber: 0.8g

Ingredients:

- 3.5 oz. of cherry tomatoes (cut them in halves)
- One medium-sized red onion (chopped finely)
- Two tablespoons each of
  - Chopped parsley
  - Extra-virgin olive oil
- One clove of garlic (halved)
- Eight units of fresh sardines (gutted and cleaned, heads should be cleaned)
- A quarter teaspoon of chili flakes
- One teaspoon of toasted cumin seeds
- Half a lemon (zested and juiced)

Method:

1. Set the temperature of the oven to 180 degrees C and preheat. Take a roasting tray and grease it lightly.

2. Take a bowl and add the tomatoes and onions in it. Add the lemon juice too and toss the veggies in the lemon juice. Now, add the zest, olive oil, chili, cumin, garlic, and parsley and toss everything once again.

3. Use pepper and salt to season the mixture. The cavity of the sardines has to be filled. Use some of the tomato and onion mixture for this purpose. Once done, place the sardines on the prepared roasting tray. Take the remaining mixture and scatter it over the sardines.

4. Roast the sardines for about 10-15 minutes, and by the end of this, they should be cooked thoroughly.

5. Serve and enjoy!

Chapter 4: Tasty Dinner Recipes

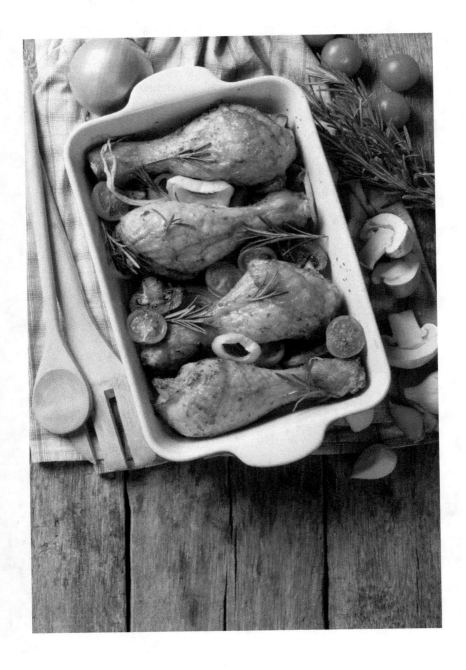

Rosemary Chicken

Total Prep & Cooking Time: 50 minutes

Yields: 4 servings

Nutrition Facts: Calories: 232 | Carbs: 3.9g | Protein: 26.7g | Fat: 11.6g | Fiber: 0.3g

Ingredients:

- Four chicken breast halves (skinless and boneless)
- One-eighth tsp. kosher salt
- One-fourth tsp. ground black pepper
- One and a half tbsps. of lemon juice
- One and a half tbsps. of Dijon mustard
- Two tbsps. of freshly minced rosemary
- Three tbsps. of olive oil
- Eight minced garlic cloves

Method:

1. At first, preheat a grill to medium-high heat. The grate needs to be lightly oiled.

2. Take a bowl and add lemon juice, mustard, rosemary, olive oil, garlic, salt, and ground black pepper. Whisk them together.

3. Take a resealable plastic bag and place the chicken breasts in it. Over the chicken, pour the garlic mixture (reserve one-eighth cup of it).

4. Seal the bag and start massaging the marinade gently into the chicken. Allow it to stand for about thirty minutes at room temperature.

5. Then on the preheated grill, place the chicken and cook for about four minutes.

6. Flip the chicken and baste it with the marinade reserved and then cook for about five minutes, until thoroughly cooked.

Finally, cover it with a foil and allow it to rest for about 2 minutes before you serve them.

Corned Beef and Cabbage

Total Prep & Cooking Time: 2 hours 35 minutes

Yields: 5 servings

Nutrition Facts: Calories: 868.8 | Carbs: 75.8g | Protein: 50.2g | Fat: 41.5g | Fiber: 14g

Ingredients:

- One big cabbage head (cut it into small wedges)
- Five peeled carrots (chopped into three-inch pieces)
- Ten red potatoes (small)
- Three pounds of corned beef brisket (along with the packet of spice)

Method:

1. At first, in a Dutch oven or a large pot, place the corned beef, and cover it with water. Then add in the spices from the packet of spices that came along with the beef. Cover the pot, bring it to a boil, and finally reduce it to a simmer. Allow it to simmer for about 2 hours and 30 minutes or until tender.

2. Add carrots and whole potatoes, and cook them until the vegetables are tender. Add the cabbage wedges and cook for another fifteen minutes. Then finally remove the meat and allow it to rest for fifteen minutes.

3. Take a bowl, place the vegetables in it, and cover it. Add broth (which is reserved in the pot) as much as you want. Then finally cut the meat against the grain.

Roasted Parsnips and Carrots

Total Prep & Cooking Time: 1 hour

Yields: 4 servings

Nutrition Facts: Calories: 112 | Carbs: 27g | Protein: 2g | Fat: 1g | Fiber: 7g

Ingredients:

- Two tbsps. of freshly minced parsley or dill
- One and a half tsp. of freshly ground black pepper
- One tbsp. kosher salt
- Three tbsps. of olive oil
- One pound of unpeeled carrots
- Two pounds of peeled parsnips

Method:

1. At first, preheat your oven to 425 degrees.

2. If the carrots and parsnips are thick, then cut them into halves lengthwise.

3. Then, slice each of them diagonally into one inch thick slices. Don't cut them too small because the vegetables will anyway shrink while you cook them.

4. Take a sheet pan, and place the cut vegetables on it.

5. Then add some olive oil, pepper, salt, and toss them nicely.

6. Roast them for about twenty to forty minutes (the roasting time depends on the size of the vegetables), accompanied by occasional tossing. Continue to roast until the carrots and parsnips become tender.

7. Finally, sprinkle some dill and serve.

Herbed Salmon

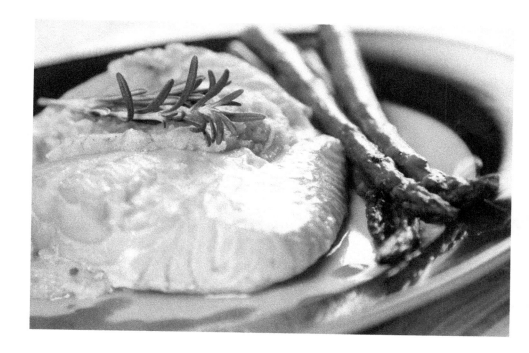

Total Prep & Cooking Time: 30 minutes

Yields: 4 servings

Nutrition Facts: Calories: 301 | Carbs: 1g | Protein: 29g | Fat: 19g | Fiber: 0g

Ingredients:

- Half a tsp. of dried thyme or two tsps. of freshly minced thyme
- Half a tsp. of pepper

- Three-fourth tsp. of salt

- One tbsp. of olive oil

- One tbsp. freshly minced rosemary or one tsp. of crushed dried rosemary.

- Four minced cloves of garlic

- Four (six ounces) fillets of salmon

Method:

1. At first, preheat your oven to 425 degrees.

2. Take a 15 by 10 by 1 inch baking pan and grease it.

3. Place the salmon on it while keeping the skin side down.

4. Combine the garlic cloves, rosemary, thyme, salt, and pepper. Spread it evenly over the salmon fillets.

5. Roast them for about fifteen to eighteen minutes until they reach your desired doneness.

Chipotle Cauliflower Tacos

Total Prep & Cooking Time: 30 minutes

Yields: 8 servings

Nutrition Facts: Calories: 440 | Carbs: 51.6g | Protein: 10.1g | Fat: 24g | Fiber: 9g

Ingredients:

For the tacos,

- Four tablespoons of avocado oil
- One head of cauliflower (large-sized, chopped into bite-sized florets)
- One cup of cilantro (freshly chopped)
- One tablespoon each of
    - Fresh lime juice
    - Maple syrup or honey
- Two tsps. of chipotle adobo sauce
- Cracked black pepper
- One teaspoon of salt
- 4-8 units of garlic cloves (freshly minced)

For the Chipotle Aioli,

- A quarter cup of chipotle adobo sauce
- Half a cup each of
    - Sour cream
    - Clean mayo

One teaspoon of sea salt

Two cloves of garlic (minced)

For serving,

- Almond flour tortillas
- Guacamole
- Almond ricotta cheese
- Sliced tomatoes, radish, and cabbage

Method:

1. Set the temperature of the oven to 425 degrees F. Now, use parchment paper to line a pan. Take the bite-sized florets of the cauliflower and spread them evenly on the pan. Use 2-4 tbsps. of avocado oil, pepper, salt, and minced garlic and drizzle it on the pan.

2. Roast the cauliflower for half an hour at 425 degrees F and halfway through the process, flip the florets.

3. When you are roasting the cauliflower, take the rest of the ingredients of the cauliflower and mix them in a bowl. Once everything has been properly incorporated, set the mixture aside.

4. Now, take another bowl and in it, add the ingredients of the chipotle aioli. Mix them and set the bowl aside.

5. If you have any other taco fixings, get them ready.

6. Once the cauliflower is ready, toss the florets in the chipotle sauce.

7. Serve the cauliflower in tortillas along with fixings of your choice and the chipotle aioli.

PART IV

In this chapter, we are going to study the details of the reset diet and what recipes you can make.

Chapter 1: How to Reset Your Body?

Created by a celebrity trainer, Harley Pasternak, the body reset diet is a famous fifteen-day eating pattern that aims to jump-start weight loss. According to Pasternak, if you experience rapid loss in weight early in a diet, you will feel more motivated to stick to that diet plan. This theory is even supported by a few scientific studies (Alice A Gibson, 2017).

The body reset diet claims to help in weight loss with light exercise and low-calorie diet plans for fifteen days. The diet is divided into 3 phases of five days each. Each phase had a particular pattern of diet and exercise routine. You need to consume food five times every day, starting from the first phase, which mostly consists of smoothies and progressing to more solid foods in the second and third phases.

The three phases of the body reset diet are:

- **Phase One** – During this stage, you are required to consume only two snacks every day and drink smoothies for breakfast, lunch, and dinner. In the case of exercise, you have to walk at least ten thousand steps per day.

- **Phase Two** – During this phase, you can eat two snacks each day, consume solid food only once, and have to replace any two meals of the day with smoothies. In case of exercise, apart from walking ten thousand steps every day, on three of the days, you also have to finish five minutes of resistance training with the help of four separate exercises.

- **Phase Three** – You can consume two snacks every day, but you have to eat two low-calorie meals and replace one of your meals with a smoothie. For exercise, you are required to walk ten thousand steps. Apart from that, you also have to finish five minutes of resistance training with the help of four separate exercises each day.

After you have finished the standard fifteen-day diet requirements, you have to keep following the meal plan you followed in the third phase. However, during this time, you are allowed to have two "free meals" twice a week in which you can consume anything you want. These "free meals" are meant as a reward so that you can avoid feeling deprived. According to Pasternak, depriving yourself of a particular food continuously can result in binge eating (Nawal Alajmi, 2016).

There is no official endpoint of the diet after the first fifteen days for losing and maintaining weight. Pasternak suggests that the habits and routines formed over fifteen days should be maintained for a lifetime.

Chapter 2: Science Behind Metabolism Reset

Several people take on a "cleanse" or "detox" diet every year to lose the extra holiday weight or simply start following healthy habits. However, some fat diet plans are often a bit overwhelming. For example, it requires a tremendous amount of self-discipline to drink only juices. Moreover, even after finishing a grueling detox diet plan, you might just go back to eating foods that are bad for you because of those days of deprivation. New studies issued in the *Medicine & Science in Sports & Exercise* shows that low-calorie diets may result in binge eating, which is not the right method for lasting weight loss.

Another research conducted by the researchers at Loughborough University showed that healthy, college-aged women who followed a calorie-restricted diet consumed an extra three hundred calories at dinner as compared to the control group who consumed three standard meals. They revealed that it was because they had lower levels of peptide YY (represses appetite) and higher levels of ghrelin (makes you hungry). They are most likely to go hog wild when you are feeling ravenous, and it's finally time to eat (Nawal Alajmi K. D.-O., 2016).

Another research published in *Cognitive Neuroscience* studied the brains of chronic dieters. They revealed that there was a weaker connection between the two regions of the brain in people who had a higher percentage of body fat. They showed that they might have an increased risk of getting obese because it's harder for them to set their temptations aside (Pin-Hao Andy Chen, 2016).

A few other studies, however, also revealed that you could increase your self-control through practice. Self-control, similar to any other kind of strength, also requires time to develop. However, you can consider focusing on a diet plan that can help you "reset" instead of putting all your efforts into developing your self-control to get healthy.

A reset is considered as a new start – one that can get your metabolism and your liver in good shape. The liver is the biggest solid organ of your body, and it's mainly responsible for removing toxins that can harm your health and well-being by polluting your system. Toxins keep accumulating in your body all the time, and even though it's the liver's job to handle this, it can sometimes get behind schedule, which can result in inflammation. It causes a lot of strain on your metabolism and results in weight gain, particularly around the abdomen. The best method to alleviate this inflammation is to follow a metabolism rest diet and give your digestive system a vacation (Olivia M. Farr, 2015).

Chapter 3: Recipes for Smoothies and Salads

If you want to lose weight and you have a particular period within which you want to achieve it, then here are some recipes that are going to be helpful.

Green Smoothie

Total Prep & Cooking Time: 2 minutes

Yields: 1 serving

Nutrition Facts: Calories: 144 | Carbs: 28.2g | Protein: 3.4g | Fat: 2.9g | Fiber: 4.8g

Ingredients:

- One cup each of
  - Almond milk
  - Raw spinach
- One-third of a cup of strawberries
- One orange, peeled

Method:

1. Add the peeled orange, strawberries, almond milk, and raw spinach in a blender and blend everything until you get a smooth paste. You can add extra water if required to achieve the desired thickness.

2. Pour out the smoothie into a glass and serve.

Strawberry Banana Smoothie

Total Prep & Cooking Time: 5 minutes

Yields: 2 servings

Nutrition Facts: Calories: 198| Carbs: 30.8g | Protein: 5.9g | Fat: 7.1g | Fiber: 4.8g

Ingredients:

- Half a cup each of
  - Milk
  - Greek yogurt
- One banana, frozen and quartered
- Two cups of fresh strawberries, halved

Method:

1. Add the milk, Greek yogurt, banana, and strawberries into a high-powered blender and blend until you get a smooth mixture.

2. Pour the smoothie equally into two separate glasses and serve.

Notes:

- *Don't add ice to the smoothie as it can make it watery very quickly. Using frozen bananas will keep your smoothie cold.*

- *As you're using bananas and strawberries, there is no need to add any artificial sweetener.*

Salmon Citrus Salad

Total Prep & Cooking Time: 20 minutes

Yields: 6 servings

Nutrition Facts: Calories: 336 | Carbs: 20g | Protein: 17g | Fat: 21g | Fiber: 5g

Ingredients:

- One pound of Citrus Salmon (slow-roasted)
- Half of an English cucumber, sliced
- One tomato (large), sliced into a quarter of an inch thick pieces
- One grapefruit, peeled and cut into segments
- Two oranges, peeled and cut into segments
- Three beets, roasted and quartered
- One avocado
- Boston lettuce leaves
- Two tablespoons of red wine vinegar
- Half of a red onion
- Flakey salt
- Aleppo pepper flakes

For the Citrus Shallot Vinaigrette,

- Five tablespoons of olive oil (extra-virgin)
- One clove of garlic, smashed
- Salt and pepper
- One and a half tablespoons of rice wine vinegar
- Two tablespoons of orange juice or fresh lemon juice

- One tablespoon of shallot, minced

Method:

For preparing the Citrus Shallot Vinaigrette:

1. Add the ingredients for the vinaigrette in a bowl and whisk them together.

2. Keep the mixture aside.

For assembling the salad,

1. Add the onions and vinegar in a small bowl and pickle them by letting them sit for about fifteen minutes.

2. In the meantime, place the lettuce leaves on the serving plate.

3. Dice the avocado in half and eliminate the pit. Then scoop the flesh and add them onto the plate. Sprinkle a dash of flakey salt and Aleppo pepper on top to season it.

4. Add the quartered beets onto the serving plate along with the grapefruit and orange segments.

5. Salt the cucumber and tomato slices lightly and add them onto the plate.

6. Then, scatter the pickled onions on top and cut the salmon into bits and add it on the plate.

7. Lastly, drizzle the Citrus Shallot Vinaigrette on top of the salad and finish off with a dash of flakey salt.

Chapter 4: Quick and Easy Breakfast and Main Course Recipes

Quinoa Salad

Total Prep & Cooking Time: 40 minutes

Yields: Eight servings

Nutrition Facts: Calories: 205 | Carbs: 25.9g | Protein: 6.1g | Fat: 9.4g | Fiber: 4.6g

Ingredients:

- One tablespoon of red wine vinegar
- One-fourth of a cup each of
  - Lemon juice (about two to three lemons)
  - Olive oil
- One cup each of
  - Quinoa (uncooked), rinsed with the help of a fine-mesh colander
  - Flat-leaf parsley (from a single large bunch), finely chopped
- Three-fourth of a cup of red onion (one small red onion), chopped
- One red bell pepper (medium-sized), chopped
- One cucumber (medium-sized), seeded and chopped
- One and a half cups of chickpeas (cooked), or One can of chickpeas (about fifteen ounces), rinsed and drained
- Two cloves of garlic, minced or pressed
- Two cups of water
- Black pepper, freshly ground
- Half a teaspoon of fine sea salt

Method:

1. Place a medium-sized saucepan over medium-high heat and add the rinsed quinoa into it along with the water. Allow the mixture to boil and then reduce the heat and simmer it. Cook for about fifteen minutes so that the quinoa has absorbed all the water. As time goes on, decrease the heat and maintain a gentle simmer. Take the saucepan away from the heat and cover it with a lid. Allow the cooked quinoa to rest for about five minutes to give it some time to increase in size.

2. Add the onions, bell pepper, cucumber, chickpeas, and parsley in a large serving bowl and mix them together. Keep the mixture aside.

3. Add the garlic, vinegar, lemon juice, olive oil, and salt in another small bowl and whisk the ingredients so that they are appropriately combined. Keep this mixture aside.

4. When the cooked quinoa has almost cooled down, transfer it to the serving bowl. Add the dressing on top and toss to combine everything together.

5. Add an extra pinch of sea salt and the black pepper to season according to your preference. Allow the salad to rest for five to ten minutes before serving it for the best results.

6. You can keep the salad in the refrigerator for up to four days. Make sure to cover it properly.

7. You can serve it at room temperature or chilled.

Notes: Instead of cooking additional quinoa, you can use about three cups of leftover quinoa for making this salad. Moreover, you can also serve this salad with fresh greens and an additional drizzle of lemon juice and olive oil. You can also add a dollop of cashew sour cream or crumbled feta cheese as a topping.

Herb and Goat Cheese Omelet

Total Prep & Cooking Time: 20 minutes

Yields: Two servings

Nutrition Facts: Calories: 233 | Carbs: 3.6g | Protein: 16g | Fat: 17.6g | Fiber: 1g

Ingredients:

- Half a cup each of
  - Red bell peppers (3 x quarter-inch), julienne-cut
  - Zucchini, thinly sliced
- Four large eggs
- Two teaspoons of olive oil, divided
- One-fourth of a cup of goat cheese (one ounce), crumbled
- Half a teaspoon of fresh tarragon, chopped
- One teaspoon each of
  - Fresh parsley, chopped
  - Fresh chives, chopped
- One-eighth of a teaspoon of salt
- One-fourth of a teaspoon of black pepper, freshly ground (divided)
- One tablespoon of water

Method:

1. Break the eggs into a bowl and add one tablespoon of water into it. Whisk them together and add in one-eighth of a teaspoon each of salt and ground black pepper.

2. In another small bowl, mix the goat cheese, tarragon, and parsley and keep it aside.

3. Place a nonstick skillet over medium heat and heat one teaspoon of olive oil in it. Add in the sliced zucchini, bell pepper, and the remaining one-eighth of a teaspoon of black pepper along with a dash of salt. Cook for about four minutes so that the bell pepper and zucchini get soft. Transfer the zucchini-bell pepper mixture onto a plate and cover it with a lid to keep it warm.

4. Add about half a teaspoon of oil into a skillet and add in half of the whisked egg into it. Do not stir the eggs and let the egg set slightly. Loosen the set edges of the omelet carefully with the help of a spatula. Tilt the skillet to move the uncooked part of the egg to the side. Keep following this method for about five seconds so that there is no more runny egg in the skillet. Add half of the crumbled goat cheese mixture evenly over the omelet and let it cook for another minute so that it sets.

5. Transfer the omelet onto a plate and fold it into thirds.

6. Repeat the process with the rest of the egg mixture, half a teaspoon of olive oil, and the goat cheese mixture.

7. Add the chopped chives on top of the omelets and serve with the bell pepper and zucchini mixture.

Mediterranean Cod

Total Prep & Cooking Time: 15 minutes

Yields: 4 servings

Nutrition Facts: Calories: 320 | Carbs: 31g | Protein: 35g | Fat: 8g | Fiber: 8g

Ingredients:

- One pound of spinach
- Four fillets of cod (almost one and a half pounds)
- Two zucchinis (medium-sized), chopped
- One cup of marinara sauce
- One-fourth of a teaspoon of red pepper, crushed
- Two cloves of garlic, chopped
- One tablespoon of olive oil
- Salt and pepper, according to taste
- Whole wheat roll, for serving

Method:

1. Place a ten-inch skillet on medium heat and add the marinara sauce and zucchini into it. Combine them together and let it simmer on medium heat.

2. Add the fillets of cod into the simmering sauce. Add one-fourth of a teaspoon each of salt and pepper too. Cover the skillet with a lid and let it cook for about seven minutes so that the cod gets just opaque throughout.

3. In the meantime, place a five-quart saucepot on medium heat and heat the olive oil in it. Add in the crushed red pepper and minced garlic. Stir and cook for about a minute.

4. Then, add in the spinach along with one-eighth of a teaspoon of salt. Cover the saucepot with a lid and let it cook for about five minutes, occasionally stirring so that the spinach gets wilted.

5. Add the spinach on the plates and top with the sauce and cod mixture and serve with the whole wheat roll.

Grilled Chicken and Veggies

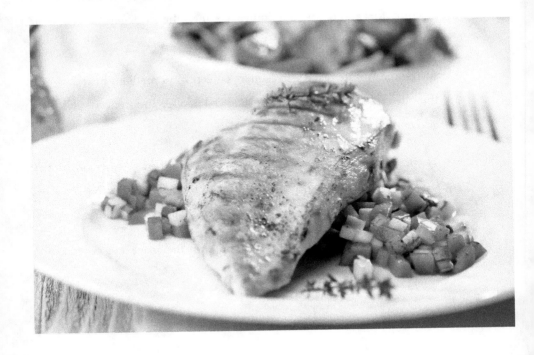

Total Prep & Cooking Time: 35 minutes

Yields: 4 servings

Nutrition Facts: Calories: 305 | Carbs: 11g | Protein: 26g | Fat: 17g | Fiber: 3g

Ingredients:

For the marinade,

- Four cloves of garlic, crushed

- One-fourth of a cup each of
  - Fresh lemon juice
  - Olive oil
- One teaspoon each of
  - Salt
  - Smoked paprika
  - Dried oregano
- Black pepper, according to taste
- Half a teaspoon of red chili flakes

For the grilling,

- Two to three zucchinis or courgette (large), cut into thin slices
- Twelve to sixteen spears of asparagus, woody sides trimmed
- Broccoli
- Two bell peppers, seeds eliminated and cut into thin slices
- Four pieces of chicken breasts (large), skinless and de-boned

Method:

1. Preheat your griddle or grill pan.

2. Sprinkle some salt on top of the chicken breasts to season them. Keep them aside to rest while you prepare the marinade.

3. For the marinade, mix all the ingredients properly.

4. Add about half of the marinade over the vegetables and the other half over the seasoned chicken breasts. Allow the marinade to rest for a couple of minutes.

5. Place the chicken pieces on the preheated grill. Grill for about five to seven minutes on each side until they are cooked according to your preference. The time on the grill depends on the thickness of the chicken breasts.

6. Remove them from the grill and cover them using a foil. Set it aside to rest and prepare to grill the vegetables in the meantime.

7. Grill the vegetables for a few minutes until they begin to char and are crispy yet tender.

8. Remove them from the grill and transfer them onto a serving plate. Serve the veggies along with the grilled chicken and add the lemon wedges on the side for squeezing.

Notes: *You can add as much or as little vegetables as you like. The vegetable amounts are given only as a guide. Moreover, feel free to replace some of them with the vegetables you like to eat.*

Stuffed Peppers

Total Prep & Cooking Time: 50 minutes

Yields: 4 servings

Nutrition Facts: Calories: 438 | Carbs: 32g | Protein: 32g | Fat: 20g | Fiber: 5g

Ingredients:

For the stuffed peppers,

- One pound of ground chicken or turkey
- Four bell peppers (large) of any color
- One and a quarter of a cups of cheese, shredded
- One and a half cups of brown rice, cooked (you can use cauliflower rice or quinoa)
- One can (about fourteen ounces) of fire-roasted diced tomatoes along with its juices
- Two teaspoons of olive oil (extra-virgin)
- One teaspoon each of
  - Garlic powder
  - Ground cumin
- One tablespoon of ground chili powder
- One-fourth of a teaspoon of black pepper
- Half a teaspoon of kosher salt

For serving,

- Sour cream or Greek yogurt

- Salsa

- Freshly chopped cilantro

- Avocado, sliced

- Freshly squeezed lemon juice

Method:

1. Preheat your oven to 375 degrees Fahrenheit.

2. Take a nine by thirteen-inch baking dish and coat it lightly with a nonstick cooking spray.

3. Take the bell peppers and slice them from top to bottom into halves. Remove the membranes and the seeds. Keep the bell peppers in the baking dish with the cut-side facing upwards.

4. Place a large, nonstick skillet on medium-high heat and heat the olive oil in it. Add in the chicken, pepper, salt, garlic powder, ground cumin, and chili powder and cook for about four minutes so that the chicken is cooked through and gets brown. Break apart the chicken while it's cooking. Drain off any excess liquid and then add in the can of diced tomatoes along with the juices. Allow it to simmer for a minute.

5. Take the pan away from the heat. Add in the cooked rice along with three-fourth of a cup of the shredded cheese and stir everything together.

6. Add this filling inside the peppers and add the remaining shredded cheese as a topping.

7. Add a little amount of water into the pan containing the peppers so that it barely covers the bottom of the pan.

8. Keep it uncovered and bake it in the oven for twenty-five to thirty-five minutes so that the cheese gets melted and the peppers get soft.

9. Add any of your favorite fixings as a topping and serve hot.

Notes:

- *For preparing the stuffed peppers ahead of time, make sure to allow the rice and chicken mixture to cool down completely before filling the peppers. You can prepare the stuffed peppers before time, and then you have to cover it with a lid and keep it in the refrigerator for a maximum of twenty-four hours before baking the peppers.*

- *If you're planning to reheat the stuffed peppers, gently reheat them in your oven or microwave. If you're using a microwave for this purpose, make sure to cut the peppers into pieces to warm them evenly.*

- *You can store any leftovers in the freezer for up to three months. Alternatively, you can keep them in the refrigerator for up to four days. Allow it to thaw in the fridge overnight.*

Brussels Sprouts With Honey Mustard Chicken

Total Prep & Cooking Time: Fifty minutes

Yields: Four servings

Nutrition Facts: Calories: 360 | Carbs: 14.5g | Protein: 30.8g | Fat: 20g | Fiber: 3.7g

Ingredients:

- One and a half pounds of Brussels sprouts, divided into two halves
- Two pounds of chicken thighs, skin-on and bone-in (about four medium-sized thighs)
- Three cloves of garlic, minced
- One-fourth of a large onion, cut into slices
- One tablespoon each of
  - Honey
  - Whole-grain mustard
  - Dijon mustard
- Two tablespoons of freshly squeezed lemon juice (one lemon)
- One-fourth of a cup plus two tablespoons of olive oil (extra-virgin)
- Freshly ground black pepper
- Kosher salt
- Non-stick cooking spray

Method:

1. Preheat your oven to 425 degrees Fahrenheit.

2. Take a large baking sheet and grease it with nonstick cooking spray. Keep it aside.

3. Add the minced garlic, honey, whole-grain mustard, Dijon mustard, one tablespoon of the lemon juice, one-fourth cup of the olive oil in a medium-sized bowl and mix them together. Add the Kosher salt and black pepper to season according to your preference.

4. Dip the chicken thighs into the sauce with the help of tongs and coat both sides. Transfer the things on the baking sheet. You can get rid of any extra sauce.

5. Mix the red onion and Brussels sprouts in a medium-sized bowl and drizzle one tablespoon of lemon juice along with the remaining two tablespoons of olive oil onto it. Toss everything together until the vegetables are adequately coated.

6. Place the red onion-Brussels sprouts mixture on the baking sheet around the chicken pieces. Ensure that the chicken and vegetables are not overlapping.

7. Sprinkle a little amount of salt and pepper on the top and keep it in the oven to roast for about thirty to thirty-five minutes so that the Brussels sprouts get crispy and the chicken has an internal temperature of 165 degrees Fahrenheit and has turned golden brown.

8. Serve hot.

Quinoa Stuffed Chicken

Total Prep & Cooking Time: 50 minutes

Yields: Four servings

Nutrition Facts: Calories: 355 | Carbs: 28g | Protein: 30g | Fat: 13g | Fiber: 4g

Ingredients:

- One and a half cups of chicken broth
- Three-fourths of a cup of quinoa (any color of your choice)
- Four chicken breasts (boneless and skinless)
- One lime, zested and one tablespoon of lime juice
- One-fourth of a cup of cilantro, chipped
- One-third of a cup of unsweetened coconut, shaved or coconut chips
- One Serrano pepper, seeded and diced
- Two cloves of garlic, minced
- Half a cup of red onion, diced
- Three-fourth of a cup of bell pepper, diced
- One tablespoon of coconut oil
- One teaspoon each of
  - Salt
  - Chili powder
  - Ground cumin

Method:

1. Preheat your oven to 375 degrees Fahrenheit.

2. Take a rimmed baking sheet and line it with parchment paper.

3. Place a medium-sized saucepan over medium-high heat and add the coconut oil in it. After it has melted, add in the Serrano peppers, garlic, red onion, and bell pepper and sauté for about one to two minutes so that they soften just a bit. Make sure that the vegetables are still bright in color. Then transfer the cooked vegetables into a bowl.

4. Add the quinoa in the empty sauce pot and increase the heat to high. Pour the chicken broth in it along with half a teaspoon of salt. Close the lid of the pot and bring it to a boil, allowing the quinoa to cook for about fifteen minutes so that the surface of the quinoa develops vent holes, and the broth has absorbed completely. Take the pot away from the heat and allow it to steam for an additional five minutes.

5. In the meantime, cut a slit along the long side in each chicken breast. It will be easier with the help of a boning knife. You are making a deep pocket in each breast, having a half-inch border around the remaining three attached sides. Keep the knife parallel to the cutting board and cut through the middle of the breast and leaving the opposite side attached. Try to cut it evenly as it's challenging to cook thick uncut portions properly in the oven. After that, add salt, cumin, and chili powder on all sides of the chicken.

6. When the quinoa has turned fluffy, add in the lime juice, lime zest, shaved coconut, and sautéed vegetables and stir them in. Taste the mixture and adjust the salt as per your preference.

7. Add the confetti quinoa mixture inside the cavity of the chicken breast. Place the stuffed breasts on the baking sheet with the quinoa facing upwards. They'll look like open envelopes.

8. Bake them in the oven for about twenty minutes.

9. Serve warm.

Kale and Sweet Potato Frittata

Total Prep & Cooking Time: 30 minutes

Yields: 4 servings

Nutrition Facts: Calories: 144 | Carbs: 10g | Protein: 7g | Fat: 9g | Fiber: 2g

Ingredients:

- Three ounces of goat cheese
- Two cloves of garlic
- Half of a red onion (small)
- Two cups each of
  o Sweet potatoes
  o Firmly packed kale, chopped
- Two tablespoons of olive oil
- One cup of half-and-half
- Six large eggs
- Half a teaspoon of pepper, freshly ground
- One teaspoon of Kosher salt

Method:

1. Preheat your oven to 350 degrees Fahrenheit.

2. Add the eggs, half-and-half, salt, and black pepper in a bowl and whisk everything together.

3. Place a ten-inch ovenproof nonstick skillet over medium heat and add one tablespoon of oil in it. Sauté the sweet potatoes in the skillet for about eight to ten minutes so that they turn soft and golden brown. Transfer them onto a plate and keep warm.

4. Next, add in the remaining one tablespoon of oil and sauté the kale along with the red onions and garlic in it for about three to four minutes so that the kale gets soft and wilted. Then, add in the whisked egg mixture evenly over the vegetables and cook for an additional three minutes.

5. Add some goat cheese on the top and bake it in the oven for ten to fourteen minutes so that it sets.

Walnut, Ginger, and Pineapple Oatmeal

Total Prep & Cooking Time: 30 minutes

Yields: 4 servings

Nutrition Facts: Calories: 323 | Carbs: 61g | Protein: 6g |Fat: 8g | Fiber: 5g

Ingredients:

- Two large eggs
- Two cups each of
  - Fresh pineapple, coarsely chopped
  - Old-fashioned rolled oats
  - Whole milk
- One cup of walnuts, chopped
- Half a cup of maple syrup
- One piece of ginger
- Two teaspoons of vanilla extract
- Half a teaspoon of salt

Method:

1. Preheat your oven to 400 degrees Fahrenheit.

2. Add the ginger, walnuts, pineapple, oats, and salt in a large bowl and mix them together. Add the mixture evenly among four ten-ounce ramekins and keep them aside.

3. Whisk the eggs along with the milk, maple syrup, and vanilla extract in a medium-sized bowl. Pour one-quarter of this mixture into each ramekin containing the oat-pineapple mixture.

4. Keep the ramekins on the baking sheet and bake them in the oven for about twenty-five minutes until the oats turn light golden brown on the top and have set properly.

5. Serve with some additional maple syrup on the side.

Caprese Salad

Total Prep & Cooking Time: 15 minutes

Yields: 4 servings

Nutrition Facts: Calories: 216 | Carbs: 4g | Protein: 13g | Fat: 16g | Fiber: 1g

Ingredients:

For the salad,

- Nine basil leaves (medium-sized)
- Eight ounces of fresh whole-milk mozzarella cheese
- Two tomatoes (medium-sized)
- One-fourth of a teaspoon of black pepper, freshly ground
- Half a teaspoon of Kosher salt, or one-fourth of a teaspoon of sea salt

For the dressing,

- One teaspoon of Dijon mustard
- One tablespoon each of
  - Balsamic vinegar
  - Olive oil

Method:

1. Add the olive oil, balsamic vinegar, and Dijon mustard into a small bowl and whisk them together with the help of a small hand whisk so that you get a smooth salad dressing. Keep it aside.

2. Cut the tomatoes into thin slices and try to get ten slices in total.

3. Cut the mozzarella into nine thin slices with the help of a sharp knife.

4. Place the slices of tomatoes and mozzarella on a serving plate, alternating and overlapping one another. Then, add the basil leaves on the top.

5. Season the salad with black pepper and salt and drizzle the prepared dressing on top.

6. Serve immediately.

One-Pot Chicken Soup

Total Prep & Cooking Time: 30 minutes

Yields: 6 servings

Nutrition Facts: Calories: 201 | Carbs: 20g | Protein: 16g | Fat: 7g | Fiber: 16g

Ingredients:

- Three cups of loosely packed chopped kale (or other greens of your choice)
- Two cups of chicken, shredded
- One can of white beans (about fifteen ounces), slightly drained
- Eight cups of broth (vegetable broth or chicken broth)
- Four cloves of garlic, minced
- One cup of yellow or white onion, diced
- One tablespoon of avocado oil (skip if you are using bacon)
- One strip of uncured bacon, chopped (optional)
- Black pepper + sea salt, according to taste

Method:

1. Place a Dutch oven or a large pot over medium heat. When it gets hot, add in the oil or bacon (optional), stirring occasionally, and allow it to get hot for about a minute.

2. Then, add in the diced onion and sauté for four to five minutes, occasionally stirring so that the onions get fragrant and translucent. Add in the minced garlic next and sauté for another two to three minutes. Be careful so as not to burn the ingredients.

3. Then, add the chicken, slightly drained white beans, and broth and bring the mixture to a simmer. Cook for about ten minutes to bring out all the flavors. Taste the mixture and add salt and pepper to season according to your preference. Add in the chopped kale in the last few minutes of cooking. Cover the pot and let it cook until the kale has wilted.

4. Serve hot.

Notes: You can store any leftovers in the freezer for up to a month. Or, you can store them in the refrigerator for a maximum of three to four days. Simply reheat on the stovetop or in the microwave and eat it later.

Chocolate Pomegranate Truffles

Total Prep & Cooking Time: 10 minutes

Yields: Twelve to Fourteen truffles

Nutrition Facts: Calories: 95 | Carbs: 26g | Protein: 1g | Fat: 2g | Fiber: 3g

Ingredients:

- One-third of a cup of pomegranate arils
- Half a teaspoon each of
  - Vanilla extract
  - Ground cinnamon
- Half a cup of ground flax seed
- Two tablespoons of cocoa powder (unsweetened)
- About one tablespoon of water
- One and a half cups of pitted Medjool dates
- One-eighth of a teaspoon of salt

Method:

1. Add the pitted dates in a food processor and blend until it begins to form a ball. Add some water and pulse again. Add in the vanilla, cinnamon, flax seeds, cocoa powder, and salt and blend until everything is combined properly.

2. Turn off the food processor and unplug it. Add in the pomegranate arils and fold them in the mixture so that they are distributed evenly.

3. Make twelve to fourteen balls using the mixture. You can create an outer coating or topping if you want by rolling the balls in finely shredded coconut or cocoa powder.

Notes: *You can store the chocolate pomegranate truffles in the fridge in an air-tight container for a maximum of three days.*

PART V

Chapter 1: Easy Recipes for Managing Kidney Problems

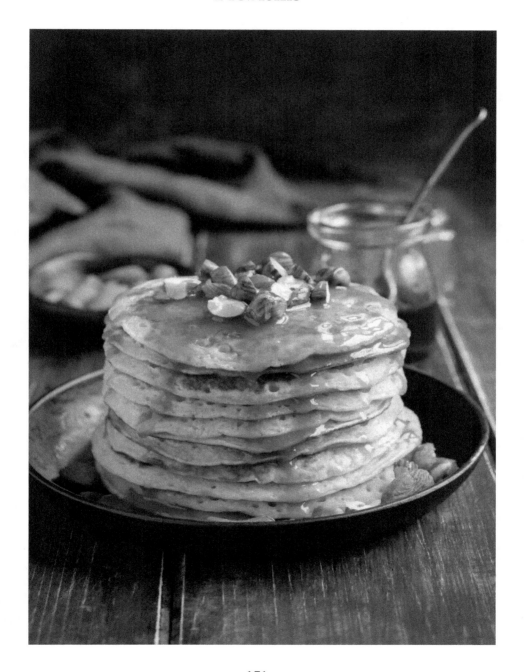

Pumpkin Pancakes

Total Prep & Cooking Time: 40 minutes

Yields: 2 servings

Nutrition Facts: Calories: 183 | Carbs: 39g | Protein: 5.4g | Fat: 1.2g | Sodium: 130mg

Ingredients:

- Two egg whites
- Two tsps. of pumpkin pie spice
- One tsp. of baking powder
- One tbsp. of brown sugar
- Three packets of Stevia
- 1.25 cups of all-purpose flour
- Two cups each of
  - Rice milk
  - Salt-free pumpkin puree

Method:

1. Start by mixing all the dry ingredients together in a bowl – baking powder, Stevia, sugar, flour, and pumpkin pie spice.

2. Now, take another bowl and, in it, mix the rice milk and pumpkin puree thoroughly.

3. In another bowl, form stiff peaks by whipping egg whites.

4. Take the mixture of dry ingredients and add them to the wet ingredients. Blend them in. Once you get a smooth mixture, add the egg whites, and whip them.

5. Grill the mixture on an oiled griddle on medium flame.

6. When you notice bubbles forming on the pancakes, you have to flip them.

7. Cook both sides of the pancakes evenly so that they turn golden brown.

Pasta Salad

Total Prep & Cooking Time: 50 minutes

Yields: 4 servings (half a cup each serving)

Nutrition Facts: Calories: 69 | Carbs: 12.5g | Protein: 2.5g | Fat: 1.3g | Sodium: 72mg

Ingredients:

- A quarter cup of olives (sliced after being pitted)
- One cup of chopped cauliflower
- Two cups of fusilli pasta (cooked)
- Half a unit each of
  - Green bell pepper (sliced)
  - Red onion (chopped)
  - Tomato (small-sized, diced)

Method:

1. Start by cooking the pasta, and for that, you have to follow the directions as mentioned on the package.

2. Now, drain the pasta. Add all the vegetables.

3. Choose any dressing of your choice, but it has to be low-fat. Toss the pasta and the veggies in the dressing.

4. Serve and enjoy!

Broccoli and Apple Salad

Total Prep & Cooking Time: 15 minutes

Yields: 8 servings (3/4 cup each serving)

Nutrition Facts: Calories: 160 | Carbs: 18g | Protein: 4g | Fat: 8g | Sodium: 63mg

Ingredients:

- Four cups of fresh florets of broccoli
- One medium-sized apple
- Half a cup each of
    - Sweetened cranberries (dried)
    - Red onion
- A quarter cup each of
    - Walnuts
    - Fresh parsley
    - Mayonnaise
- Two tbsps. each of
    - Apple cider vinegar
    - Honey
- A three-fourth cup of plain Greek yogurt (low-fat)

Method:

1. Prepare the broccoli florets by cutting into bite-sized chunks. Trim them properly. Take the apple and cut into small pieces as well but in the unpeeled state. Prepare the parsley by chopping them coarsely.

2. Now, take a large-sized bowl and add the mayonnaise, yogurt, vinegar, honey, and parsley. Whisk them together.

3. Take the remaining ingredients and add them too. Make sure they are evenly coated with the yogurt mixture. Once prepared, keep the salad in the refrigerator because it is best served when chilled. It allows the flavors to combine properly. Before serving, stir the salad.

Notes:

- *You can use your favorite type of apple.*

- *If you want, you can sprinkle some more parsley on top just before serving.*

Pineapple Frangelico Sorbet

Total Prep & Cooking Time: 2 hours 10 minutes

Yields: 4 servings

Nutrition Facts: Calories: 119 | Carbs: 28g | Protein: 1g | Fat: 0.2g | Sodium: 2.4mg

Ingredients:

- Two tsps. of Stevia
- One tbsp. of Frangelico (keep two tsps. extra)
- Half a cup of unsweetened pineapple juice
- Two cups of pineapple (fresh)

Method:

1. Take all the ingredients in the container of the blender and process them until you get a smooth mixture.

2. Then, take this mixture and divide it into ice cubes. Keep it in the refrigerator and allow it to freeze.

3. When you find that the mixture has frozen, take them out and blend them in the food processor again. This process will give you a fluffy texture.

4. Before you serve, refreeze the sorbet.

Egg Muffins

Total Prep & Cooking Time: 45 minutes

Yields: 8 servings

Nutrition Facts: Calories: 154 | Carbs: 3g | Protein: 12g | Fat: 10g | Sodium: 155mg

Ingredients:

- Half an lb. of ground pork
- Half a tsp. of herb seasoning blend of your choice
- A quarter tsp. of salt
- Eight eggs (large-sized)
- A quarter tsp. each of
  - Onion powder
  - Garlic powder
  - Poultry seasoning
- One cup each of
  - Onion
  - Bell peppers (A mixture of orange, yellow, and red)

Method:

1. Set the oven temperature to 350 degrees F and use cooking spray to coat a muffin tin of regular size.

2. Prepare the onions and bell peppers by dicing them finely.

3. Take a bowl and in it, combine the following ingredients – garlic powder, poultry seasoning, pork, onion powder, and herb seasoning blend. Form the sausage by combining all of this properly.

4. Now cook the sausage in a non-stick skillet. Once it has been appropriately cooked, drain the sausage.

5. Use salt and milk substitute/milk to beat the eggs in a bowl. In it, add the veggies and the sausage mix.

6. Take the prepared muffin tin and pour the egg mixture into it. You have to leave enough space for the muffins so that they can rise. Bake them for about 20-22 minutes.

Notes: *If there are extra muffins, then you can have them as a quick breakfast the next day, and you simply have to reheat them for about 40 seconds.*

Linguine With Broccoli, Chickpeas, and Ricotta

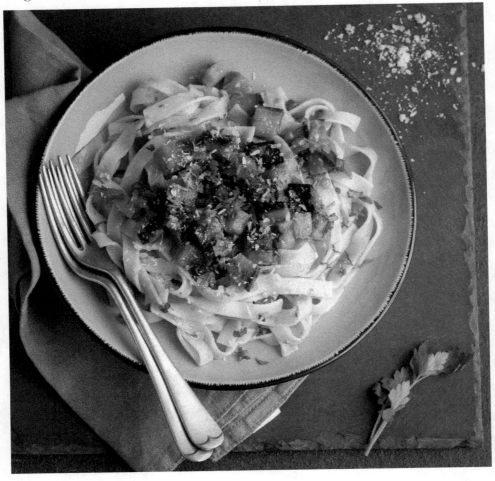

Total Prep & Cooking Time: 1 hour 5 minutes

Yields: 4 servings

Nutrition Facts: Calories: 404 | Carbs: 49.8g | Protein: 13.2g | Fat: 17.5g | Sodium: 180.4mg

Ingredients:

- Eight ounces of ricotta cheese that have been kept at room temperature
- A bunch of Tuscan kale (chopped into bite-sized chunks and stemmed)
- One-third cup of extra-virgin olive oil
- A pinch of black pepper
- Two cloves of garlic (sliced thinly)
- Fourteen ounces of chickpeas (rinsed after draining)
- Twelve ounces of spaghetti or linguine pasta
- A pinch of kosher salt
- One lemon
- Half a teaspoon of red pepper flakes
- Two tablespoons of unsalted butter
- To taste – Flaky sea salt

Method:

1. Take a large pot and add water to it. Add salt and bring the water to a boil. Cook the pasta by following the directions mentioned on the package. They must be perfectly al dente. Once the pasta is done, you have to drain it but, at the same time, reserve half a cup of the cooking water.

2. Heat the broiler and adjust the rack. Toss the following ingredients together in a bowl – garlic, chickpeas, broccoli, one-third cup of oil, and

red pepper flakes. Everything should become evenly coated. Use pepper and salt to season the mixture.

3. Take a sheet pan and spread the mixture out on it evenly.

4. Take the kale and add it to the previous bowl you used. Toss it again along with the remaining oil, if any. If you need it, then you can drizzle some more oil on top. Spread the kale in a second sheet pan in an even layer.

5. You have to take one sheet at a time while working. Broil the chickpeas and broccoli and halfway through the process, toss them. The broccoli should become charred and tender, and the chickpeas should be toasty. It will take about seven minutes. Then, broil the kale too for about five minutes, and they should become crispy.

6. Take the lemon, zest it, and then cut it into two halves. Take one half and form four wedges out of it. The juice of the lemon will have to be squeezed out on the roasted veggies and then use pepper and salt to season.

7. Place the pasta back in the pot. Take the pasta water you had earlier reserved and add it to the pasta and the lemon zest, butter, and ricotta. Keep tossing so that everything is well incorporated. Now, add the roasted veggies too. If you need, add some more pasta water while tossing.

8. Now, your linguine is done, and you have to divide it among four bowls—season with pepper and flaky sea salt. Squeeze a few drops of lemon on top and serve. If you want, drizzle some more oil before serving.

Ground Beef Soup

Total Prep & Cooking Time: 35 minutes

Yields: 6 servings

Nutrition Facts: Calories: 222 | Carbs: 19g | Protein: 20g | Fat: 8g | Sodium: 170mg

Ingredients:

- Half a cup of onion
- One tbsp. of sour cream
- Three cups of mixed vegetables (frozen, peas, green beans, corn, and carrots)
- One-third cup of uncooked white rice
- Two cups of water
- One cup of beef broth (reduced-sodium variety)
- One tsp. of browning sauce and seasoning of your choice
- Two tsps. of lemon pepper seasoning of your choice
- One lb. of ground beef (lean)

Method:

1. Prepare the onion by chopping them thoroughly. Then, take a large-sized saucepan and, in it, brown the onion and ground beef together. Drain the juices and excess fat.

2. Add the browning sauce and seasonings. Then, add the mixed veggies, rice, water, and beef broth and mix everything together.

3. Bring the mixture to a boil after placing it on high flame. Once the mixture starts boiling, reduce the flame to medium-low and cover the saucepan. Allow it to simmer and cook it for half an hour.

4. Once done, remove the pan from the flame and add the sour cream. Stir it in and serve.

Apple Oatmeal Crisp

Total Prep & Cooking Time: 40 minutes

Yields: 8 servings

Nutrition Facts: Calories: 297 | Carbs: 42g | Protein: 3g | Fat: 13g | Sodium: 95mg

Ingredients:

- A three-quarter cup of brown sugar
- Half a cup of butter
- One tsp. of cinnamon
- Half a cup of all-purpose flour
- Five apples (if possible, then Granny Smith ones)
- One cup of whole oatmeal

Method:

1. Set the temperature of the oven to 350 degrees F and preheat. Peel the apples, core them, and then cut them into slices.

2. Take a bowl and then mix the following ingredients in it together – brown sugar, oatmeal, cinnamon, and flour.

3. Use a pastry cutter to cut the butter into the oatmeal and make sure they are well blended.

4. Take a baking pan of 9 by 9 inches in size and place the sliced apples in it.

5. Take the oatmeal mixture and sprinkle it on top of the apples.

6. Bake the mixture for about thirty to thirty-five minutes.

Chapter 2: Weekend Recipes for Renal Diet

Hawaiian Chicken Salad Sandwich

Total Prep & Cooking Time: 10 minutes + chilling

Yields: 4 servings

Nutrition Facts: Calories: 349 | Carbs: 24g | Protein: 22g | Fat: 17g | Sodium: 398mg

Ingredients:

- One cup of pineapple tidbits
- Two cups of cooked chicken
- One-third cup of carrots
- Half a cup each of
  - Green bell pepper
  - Mayonnaise (low-fat)
- Four units of flatbread
- Half a tsp. of black pepper

Method:

1. Take the cooked chicken and chop it into bite-sized pieces.

2. Prepare the pineapple by draining it and then shred the carrots and chop the bell pepper.

3. Take all the ingredients in a medium-sized bowl and mix them well.

4. Refrigerate the mixture until it is thoroughly chilled.

5. Before serving, spread the chicken on the flatbread's open surface, or if you prefer it wrapped, you can use a tortilla too.

Apple Puffs

Total Prep & Cooking Time: 1 hour 20 minutes

Yields: 12 servings

Nutrition Facts: Calories: 156 | Carbs: 22g | Protein: 1.5g | Fat: 7.3g | Sodium: 176mg

Ingredients:

- Eight ounces of puff dough sheets
- One can (21 oz.) of apple pie filling
- Half a tsp. of rum extract
- One tsp. each of
  - Powdered sugar
  - Baking soda
  - Ground cinnamon

Method:

1. First, you have to thaw the puff dough sheets at room temperature, and it will take you approximately 1 hour.

2. Set the temperature of the oven to 400 degrees F and preheat.

3. Take a bowl, and in it, add the apple pie filling. If you have already sliced the apples, then you can form thirds from them now. Mix the rum extract and cinnamon with the apples.

4. Once the dough has been completely thawed, take one of the sheets and cut nine equal squares from it. Take the other sheet, and you will need only one-third of it to cut another three such squares.

5. Now, take the muffin tin and place the squares in each of the tins. In each of these squares, spoon some of the apple mixture.

6. Bake the preparation in the preheated oven for fifteen minutes, and they should become golden brown in color.

7. Once done, remove the puffs from the muffin tins and before serving, sprinkle some powdered sugar on top of each apple puff. Serve them warm.

Creamy Orzo and Vegetables

Total Prep & Cooking Time: 30 minutes

Yields: 6 servings

Nutrition Facts: Calories: 176 | Carbs: 25g | Protein: 10g | Fat: 4g | Sodium: 193mg

Ingredients:

- Half a cup of frozen green peas
- One tsp. of curry powder
- One carrot (medium-sized)
- One zucchini (small-sized)
- One onion (small-sized)
- One clove of garlic
- Three cups of chicken broth (low-sodium variety)
- Two tbsps. each of
  - Olive oil
  - Fresh parsley
- A quarter tsp. of black pepper
- A quarter cup of Parmesan cheese (freshly grated)
- One cup of cooked orzo pasta
- A quarter tsp. of salt

Method:

1. Start by preparing the veggies. Chop the zucchini and onion. Chop the garlic finely. Then, take the carrots and shred them.

2. Place a large-sized skillet on the oven over medium flame. Heat olive oil in the skillet. Sauté the following ingredients in it for about five minutes – carrots, zucchini, onion, and garlic.

3. After that, add the curry powder to the mixture. Season with salt and then add the chicken broth. Bring the mixture to a boil.

4. Now, add the cooked orzo pasta and keep stirring until the mixture starts boiling. Cover the skillet and allow the mixture to simmer. Keep stirring from time to time and cook the pasta for another 10 minutes. By this time, the pasta will become al dente, and the liquid will be absorbed.

5. Add the chopped parsley, cheese, and the frozen peas into the pasta. Keep heating until the vegetables are sufficiently hot, and if you want to enhance the creaminess, then you can add some more broth—season with pepper.

Minestrone Soup

Total Prep & Cooking Time: 45 minutes

Yields: 4 servings

Nutrition Facts: Calories: 144 | Carbs: 21.9g | Protein: 5.9g | Fat: 4.3g | Sodium: 55.1mg

Ingredients:

- Four cups of low-sodium chicken broth (low-fat)
- One carrot (large-sized)
- One and a half cups of dry macaroni (elbow-shaped)
- 14 oz. of tomatoes (diced, without any salt content)
- Two stalks of celery
- Two garlic cloves
- Half a cup of zucchini (freshly chopped)
- One teaspoon each of
  - Dried basil
  - Dried oregano
  - Freshly ground black pepper
- Half an onion (large-sized)
- One can of green snap beans (without any salt content)
- Two tbsps. of olive oil

Method:

1. Prepare the veggies by dicing zucchini, garlic, and onion. Then, take the carrots and shred them. Either use fresh green beans or canned ones, but you have to cut them into pieces of half an inch size.

2. Take a Dutch oven or a large pot and place it on medium flame—heat olive oil in the pot. Add the diced onions in the pot as well and then cook them for a couple of minutes until they become translucent.

3. Add zucchini, carrot, celery, and garlic, and if you are using fresh green beans, then add them too. Cook the vegetables for about five minutes and they will become tender.

4. Add black pepper, oregano, basil, and if you are using canned beans, then add them now.

5. Add the chicken broth and the diced tomatoes and keep stirring.

6. Bring the mixture to a boil and once it starts boiling, allow the mixture to simmer for about ten minutes.

7. Add the pasta and cook them for an additional ten minutes by following the directions mentioned on the package.

8. Before serving, garnish the pasta with fresh basil on top. Serve into bowls and enjoy!

Frosted Grapes

Total Prep & Cooking Time: 1 hour 5 minutes

Yields: 10 servings (serving size – half a cup)

Nutrition Facts: Calories: 88 | Carbs: 21g | Protein: 1g | Fat: 0g | Sodium: 41mg

Ingredients:

- Three oz. of flavored gelatin
- Five cups of seedless grapes

Method:

1. De-steam the seedless grapes after you have washed them. After that, let them be but make sure they are slightly damp.

2. In a large-sized bowl, add the dry gelatin mix. Remember that you shouldn't be pouring in water.

3. Add these damp grapes into the bowl, and in order to coat them uniformly, toss them well.

4. Now, take a baking sheet, and place these grapes on the sheet in an even layer.

5. Freeze them for 1 hour and then serve chilled.

Notes: *The flavor of the gelatin you use can be adjusted as per your choice. If you want to decrease the carbs, then use gelatin that is sugar-free.*

Yogurt and Fruit Salad

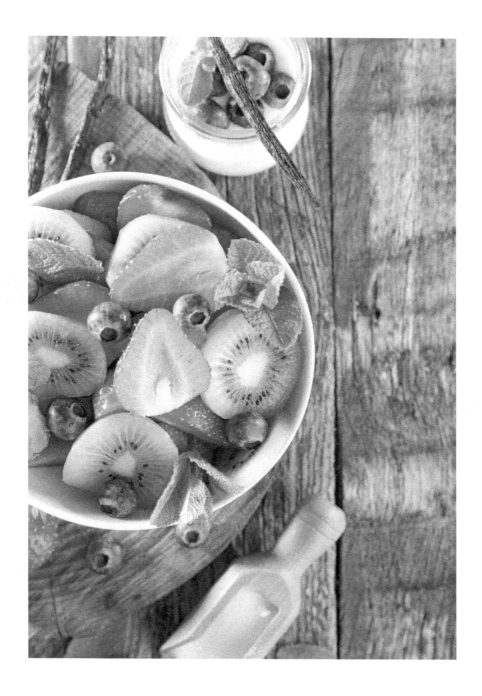

Total Prep & Cooking Time: 2 hours 20 minutes

Yields: 4 servings

Nutrition Facts: Calories: 99 | Carbs: 22g | Protein: 2.6g | Fat: 0.7g | Sodium: 12mg

Ingredients:

- One-third cup of dried cranberries
- Half a cup of pineapple chunks (fresh)
- Six strawberries (large-sized)
- Six ounces of Greek yogurt (strawberry flavored)
- Four ounces of mandarin oranges (drained, light syrup)
- Ten green grapes
- One apple (with skin, medium-sized)

Method:

1. Wash the strawberries, grapes, and apples. After that, pat them dry.

2. Slice the apples and chop them into bite-sized chunks.

3. Then, take the strawberries and slice them as well.

4. Mix the following ingredients together – yogurt, dried cranberries, pineapple, Mandarin oranges, grapes, and apples.

5. Keep the mixture covered and put it in the refrigerator for two hours.

6. Before serving, garnish the preparation with sliced strawberries.

Beet and Apple Juice Blend

Total Prep & Cooking Time: 5 minutes

Yields: 2 servings

Nutrition Facts: Calories: 53 | Carbs: 13g | Protein: 1g | Fat: 0g | Sodium: 66mg

Ingredients:

- A quarter cup of parsley
- Half a beet (medium-sized)
- Half an apple (medium-sized)
- One carrot (fresh, medium-sized)
- One stalk of celery

Method:

1. Process the following ingredients together in a juicer – parsley, celery, carrot, beet, and apple.

2. Take the mixture and pour it into two small glasses. You can either keep the juice in the refrigerator to chill or have it right away.

Notes: *Even though juices are healthy, for kidney patients, you have to be careful so that you don't increase your potassium intake too much.*

Baked Turkey Spring Rolls

Total Prep & Cooking Time: 1 hour 30 minutes

Yields: 8 servings (per serving – 2 spring rolls)

Nutrition Facts: Calories: 197 | Carbs: 9.6g | Protein: 23.3g | Fat: 7.3g | Sodium: 82.2mg

Ingredients:

- 2.5 cups of coleslaw mix
- Two tsps. of freshly ground black pepper
- Twenty ounces of turkey breast (ground)
- Two tbsps. each of
  - Vegetable oil
  - Minced cilantro
- One tbsp. each of
  - Sesame oil
  - Balsamic vinegar
- Two tsps. of freshly ground black pepper
- Sixteen pastry wrappers (frozen spring roll wraps)
- Cooking spray

Method:

1. Set the temperature of the oven to 400 degrees F and preheat.

2. Take the spring roll wrappers out from the freezer so that they can stay under room temperature. Thawing should be done at least half an hour before preparation.

3. Now, take a bowl, and in it, mix the following ingredients with the raw turkey – minced cilantro, sesame oil, and balsamic vinegar.

4. Take a large-sized skillet, and in it, pour two tbsps. of vegetable oil. Put the skillet on medium-high flame and preheat. Add the ground turkey

into the skillet and crumble it by stirring. To cook the turkey properly, you have to keep sautéing the mixture.

5. Then, you have to add the mixture of coleslaw to the turkey and keep cooking for another five minutes. Season with freshly ground black pepper – two tsps. should be enough. Mix everything properly.

6. Once done, remove the skillet from the flame. Use a strainer to drain any remaining liquid.

7. Take one spring roll wrapper and near one corner of it – add the filling diagonally. You can take three tbsps. of filling for one roll. There should be adequate space left on both sides. Fold one side towards the inside and do the same with the other side. Roll them and make sure the sights have been tucked in properly. Use water to moisten one of the sides of the wrapper because this helps to seal properly.

8. Take the remaining wrappers and follow the same steps with them.

9. Use non-stick cooking spray to coat the baking pan's base and then place the spring rolls in it. Place the pan in the oven, and it should be complete in half an hour when given at 400 degrees F.

10. You can also serve the rolls with a sweet chili sauce, but this has not been included in the nutrition facts.

Crab-Stuffed Celery Logs

Total Prep & Cooking Time: 10 minutes

Yields: 4 servings

Nutrition Facts: Calories: 34 | Carbs: 2g | Protein: 2g | Fat: 2g | Sodium: 94mg

Ingredients:

- Two tsps. of mayonnaise
- One tbsp. of red onion
- A quarter cup of crab meat
- Four ribs or celery (approx. eight inches in size)
- A quarter tsp. of paprika
- Half a tsp. of lemon juice

Method:

1. Take the celery ribs and trim the ends. Prepare the crab meat by draining it and then use two forks to flake the meat. Chop the onion and mince it thoroughly.

2. Take a small-sized bowl and in it, add the lemon juice, mayonnaise, onion, and crab meat and combine them properly.

3. Take a whole tablespoon full of the mixture and fill the celery rib with it.

4. Each rib of celery has to be cut into three equal pieces.

5. Sprinkle some paprika on top of each of these celery logs.

Couscous Salad

Total Prep & Cooking Time: 50 minutes

Yields: 4 servings (half a cup per serving)

Nutrition Facts: Calories: 151 | Carbs: 28.7g | Protein: 4.9g | Fat: 2.5g | Sodium: 14.3mg

Ingredients:

- One teaspoon each of
  - Dried oregano
  - Allspice
- Two lemons (juiced)
- One tbsp. each of
  - Olive oil
  - Minced garlic
- Half a cup each of
  - Red bell pepper (chopped)
  - Yellow bell pepper (chopped)
  - Carrots (chopped)
  - Frozen corn
- One cup each of
  - Dry couscous
  - Whole sugar snap peas
- Three peeled cucumbers (large-sized)

Method:

1. Follow the package instructions to prepare the couscous. After that, allow it to chill.

2. Take a large bowl and mix the following ingredients: cucumbers, couscous, snow peas, carrots, corn, yellow pepper, and red pepper.

3. Take another bowl of small size and, in it, whisk the following ingredients together – dried oregano, allspice, lemon juice, olive oil, and minced garlic.

4. Combine everything and serve it chilled.

Chapter 3: One-Week Meal Plan

Day 1

Breakfast – Pumpkin Pancakes

Lunch – Ground Beef Soup

Snacks – Frosted Grapes

Dinner – Pasta Salad

Day 2

Breakfast – Yogurt and Fruit Salad

Lunch – Broccoli and Apple Salad

Snacks – Apple Puffs

Dinner – Baked Turkey Spring Rolls

Day 3

Breakfast – Egg Muffins

Lunch – <u>Minestrone Soup</u>

Snacks – <u>Crab-Stuffed Celery Logs</u>

Dinner – <u>Hawaiian Chicken Salad Sandwich</u>

Day 4

Breakfast – <u>Yogurt and Fruit Salad</u>

Lunch – <u>Pasta Salad</u>

Snacks – <u>Apple Puffs</u>

Dinner – <u>Linguine with Broccoli, Chickpeas, and Ricotta</u>

Day 5

Breakfast – <u>Beet and Apple Juice Blend</u>

Lunch – <u>Ground Beef Soup</u>

Snacks – <u>Frosted Grapes</u>

Dinner – <u>Baked Turkey Spring Rolls</u>

Day 6

Breakfast – Pumpkin Pancakes

Lunch – Creamy Orzo and Vegetables

Snacks – Pineapple Frangelico Sorbet

Dinner – Couscous Salad

Day 7

Breakfast – Egg Muffins

Lunch – Broccoli and Apple Salad

Snacks – Pineapple Frangelico Sorbet

Dinner – Ground Beef Soup

Chapter 4: Avoiding Dialysis and Taking the Right Supplements

Even though getting diagnosed with chronic kidney disease (CKD) might appear scary, you can take certain steps to prolong your kidney function and delay the onset of dialysis if you catch the disease in its early stages. Some of the main causes of CKD in Americans are high blood pressure and diabetes. In order to prolong kidney function, these diseases should be controlled.

Steps to Avoid Dialysis and Prolong Kidney Function.

There are steps an individual could take to prolong kidney function regardless of how the individual developed CKD.

- **Following a renal diet** – The main aim of a pre-dialysis diet is to maintain optimum nutrition. A renal diet is one that has a low content of protein, phosphorus, and sodium and emphasizes the importance of limiting the intake of fluids and consuming high-quality protein. It's essential to consult your dietician for individualized nutrition counseling. Several doctors believe that the progression of kidney diseases can be slowed down by following a renal diet.

- **Reduce the intake of salt** – Consuming an excess amount of salt with your foods is linked with high blood pressure.

- **Exercise regularly** – Exercises like running, walking, and swimming can help maintain a healthy weight, manage diabetes and high blood pressure, and decrease stress.

- **Reduce stress** – Decreasing stress and anxiety can lower your blood pressure, which in turn can be beneficial for your kidneys.

- **Don't smoke** – Smoking decreases the flow of blood to your kidneys. It decreases kidney function in both people with or without diseases.

- **Limit alcohol intake** – Alcohol consumption can increase your blood pressure. The excess calories can also make you gain weight.

- **Drink enough water** – Your kidneys can be damaged by dehydration, decreasing blood flow to the kidneys. However, follow your nutritionist's guidelines regarding fluid intake because regular fluid intake can also increase the build-up of fluid in your body, which can become dangerous for patients in the later stages of CKD.

- **Control your blood pressure** – High blood pressure can increase your risk of kidney failure and heart diseases.

- **Control your blood sugar** – The risk of kidney failure and heart diseases are increased due to diabetes.

- **Maintain a healthy weight** – The risk of kidney-related conditions like high blood pressure and diabetes can be increased because of obesity.

Even though CKD cannot be reversed, appropriate treatment can slow down its progression. See your doctor regularly to monitor your kidney function and slow the progression of kidney failure.

Supplements to Look Out for

The dietary requirements of people who are suffering from any sort of kidney problems are not always the same. Someone might need extra calories and proteins, whereas others might need fewer amounts of such nutrients. Thus, a professional healthcare provider is the best person who can assist and guide you for choosing the perfect supplements necessary for your kidney disease. Special supplements meant for keeping the kidney safe are available in various sizes, shapes, flavors, and forms. It is always necessary to consult a healthcare practitioner before consuming any nutritional supplement related to the kidney.

Individuals who are suffering from chronic kidney disease (CKD) require certain water-soluble vitamins in higher quantities. Here you will get to know about some of the supplements that are meant for dealing with kidney problems.

- **Vitamin B1 or Thiamin -** It looks after the proper functioning of the nervous system. Thiamin also helps the cells in producing the required amount of energy from carbohydrates. People with chronic kidney disease are recommended to intake 1.5mg of this water-soluble vitamin supplement per day.

- **Vitamin B2 or Riboflavin -** Vitamin B2 supports healthy skin as well as normal vision. People who are fighting against CKD and are also following a special low-protein diet might consume 1.8mg of Riboflavin supplement each day. Those of you who have a low appetite and are pursuing dialysis might take 1.1 to 1.3mg of vitamin B2 supplements per day.

- **Vitamin B6 -** This effective water-soluble vitamin helps produce proteins that are further used for making cells. Patients of CKD who are under dialysis treatment might consume 10mg of this supplement each day. Those who are non-dialysis patients are recommended to intake 5mg vitamin B6 supplements every day.

- **NAC -** NAC or N-acetylcysteine is an essential amino acid that generally targets the oxygen radicals. Various findings and researches suggest that NAC supplementation is beneficial for hemodialysis patients. NAC supplement decreases oxidative stress as well as improves results of uremic anemia, which is a problem of CKD.

- **ALA -** The antioxidant Alpha lipoic acid might prove helpful in treating certain complications of kidney disease. Supplementation of ALA enhances the action of a few antioxidant enzymes. Such enzymes protect against oxidative disorders and stress.

- **Vitamin B12 -** Vitamin B12 maintains the nerve cells and, in association with folate, produces red blood cells. Both dialysis and non-dialysis CKD patients are recommended to intake 2-3 mg of this supplement per day. Its deficiency can result in permanent nerve damage.

Supplements for kidney problems are better to consume only if it is approved or prescribed by your doctor.

CPSIA information can be obtained
at www.ICGtesting.com
Printed in the USA
BVHW040931210920
589272BV00011B/885